Praise for
mom energy

"Mom Energy offers a great gift to moms everywhere—tools to help end our exhaustion! Ashley and Kathy offer real-life tips and strategies for developing self-replenishing energy and balance. Thanks, ladies!"

— **Cindy Crawford**

"Mom Energy is a must-read—not just for all moms, but for all women. This book will change not only your energy but your life."

— **KaDee Strickland**, actress, ABC's hit series *Private Practice*

"A superb book! Mom Energy combines cutting-edge science with common sense. Far surpassing the norm for 'how-to' books, Koff and Kaehler combine forces to deliver a book that truly integrates effective dietary and lifestyle programs for better health. I'd recommend it to any mom who is perpetually running on fumes; this book may be her ticket to revitalization."

— **Gerard E. Mullin, M.D.**, associate professor of medicine, Johns Hopkins University School of Medicine and author of *The Inside Tract*

"Read this book. I wish I had it when my girls were young . . . it's inspiring! Tune in to your Mom Energy."

— **Mariel Hemingway**, actress and author

"I am so glad I read Mom Energy as a soon-to-be-mom! I encourage moms with children of all ages—and expectant moms, too—to pick up this book. Really, any woman will benefit, because what woman doesn't need more energy in her life? This book is the answer to all of your energy needs!"

— **Emily Deschanel**, actress, FOX's hit series *Bones*

"Mom Energy recognizes that health is all about balance. This book will help fuel our world's most precious resource—moms!"

— **Rachel Lincoln Sarnoff**, executive director/CEO of Healthy Child Healthy World

"Mom Energy is every mother's dream: a true time-saver, body-saver, and life-saver! Brava! From one especially grateful mom."

— **Mayim Bialik, Ph.D.**, actress, CBS's hit series *The Big Bang Theory*

"As a working mother constantly on the go, I applaud Koff and Kaehler for providing timeless nutrition tips and fitness workouts that I can immediately incorporate into my daily routines."

— **Melissa Rivers**, host, author, and mom

mom energy

mom energy

A SIMPLE PLAN TO LIVE FULLY CHARGED

From the Experts Who Coach
Hollywood's Most Celebrated Moms

ASHLEY KOFF, R.D.
KATHY KAEHLER

HAY HOUSE, INC.
Carlsbad, California • New York City
London • Sydney • Johannesburg
Vancouver • Hong Kong • New Delhi

Published and distributed in the United States by: Hay House, Inc.: www.hay house.com • **Published and distributed in Australia by:** Hay House Australia Pty. Ltd.: www.hayhouse.com.au • **Published and distributed in the United Kingdom by:** Hay House UK, Ltd.: www.hayhouse.co.uk • **Published and distributed in the Republic of South Africa by:** Hay House SA (Pty), Ltd.: www.hayhouse.co.za • **Distributed in Canada by:** Raincoast: www.raincoast.com • **Published in India by:** Hay House Publishers India: www.hayhouse.co.in

Cover design: Lisa Fyfe • *Interior design:* Charles McStravick

Library of Congress Cataloging-in-Publication Data

Koff, Ashley.
  Mom energy : a simple plan to live fully charged / Ashley Koff and Kathy Kaehler. -- 1st ed.
    p. cm.
  ISBN 978-1-4019-3151-3 (hardback) -- ISBN 978-1-4019-3153-7 (digital) 1. Women--Health and hygiene. 2. Physical fitness. 3. Motherhood. I. Kaehler, Kathy. II. Title.
  RA778.K72237 2011
  613'.04244--dc23
                              2011019362

Hardcover ISBN: 978-1-4019-3151-3
Digital ISBN: 978-1-4019-3153-7

14 13 12 11   4 3 2 1
1st edition, September 2011

Printed in the United States of America

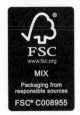

TO MOTHERS
EVERYWHERE

In the 21st century the energy crisis is getting personal.
It's not only about the environment. Just ask any mom!
The most precious and scarcest resource of all is
"mom energy." We're committed to helping
women turn this energy crisis around—
one mom at a time.

— ASHLEY AND KATHY

CONTENTS

Introduction: Solving the Real Energy Crisis of the 21st Century xi

PART I: BEFORE YOU GET STARTED

CHAPTER 1: Master Your Body's Native Energy Language 3

CHAPTER 2: Determine Your Profile: Put Your Energy to the Test . . 29

PART II: REORGANIZE

CHAPTER 3: Time Warp: Get More Done in Less Time 45

CHAPTER 4: The Energy Exchange Part 1:
Ditch Energy Drainers in Your Diet 63

CHAPTER 5: The Energy Exchange Part 2: Choose
Energy Solutions in the Marketplace 91

PART III: REHABILITATE

CHAPTER 6: Rehabilitate Your Body:
Relieve Advanced Imbalances 129

CHAPTER 7: Reboot: Cleanse and Supplement 161

PART IV: RECHARGE

CHAPTER 8: Make Magic with Movement:
Bring Exercise into Your Day 183

CHAPTER 9: Refuel: Bring Sleep into Your Night 203

CHAPTER 10: Have Fun: Learn the Power of Play 215

Conclusion: The Choice Is Yours 237
Appendix: The Whole-Body List of Top Exercises 239
Acknowledgments 247
About the Authors 249

Solving the Real Energy Crisis of the 21st Century

mom (mäm): n. the woman for whom energy demands consistently exceed her reserves.

en–er–gy ('en-ər-jē): n. the strength and vitality required for life.

Mom En–er–gy: n. the solution to "mom depletion."

It's nearly midnight and you're still in the kitchen getting ready for tomorrow; in the back of your mind is the urge to log back on to the computer to deal with e-mails marked high-priority (!), a few RSVPs you've been avoiding (!!), and late bills (!!!). The house is finally quiet but you know that the morning alarm will ring soon enough. Too soon, in fact. If a genie were to emerge and grant you three wishes, they'd all be the same: more energy, more energy, more energy. (Okay, so maybe losing 15 pounds and your crow's-feet are also on that list, but we'll get to that.)

Never before has balancing the competing demands of workplace, home, and health been more grueling—or more essential. And, let's face it, we don't know any mother who isn't taking on more than she ever intended to when she said "I do" to having children. Every mom we know has more to do in a day than the time in which to do it.

From the very second you got pregnant, your baby took energy from you, and you've had to share that energy ever since. Now you're the CEO of a family that needs and relies on you, that expects you to be superhuman and somehow conjure the energy to do anything and everything. Your own expectations of yourself are even more rigorous and demanding because you really do want to be the EveryMom—the woman who conquers all with aplomb.

But a big part of you yearns for the magic potion that will infuse you with an eternal source of high, natural, and radiant energy. All year long you've been reading about the latest recovery idea for the economy, and you wonder, *Where's my recovery?*

Well, here's your stimulus package. And this one will last a lot longer than any getting doled out in Washington, D.C.

Two Women on a Mission

But before we lay out the details of our plan, let us tell you a little about ourselves. We've been working in the trenches of fitness and nutrition for years, pretty much our entire professional lives; and between us, we cover every angle of the mom-depletion phenomenon. We've worked with hundreds of women—celebrity and civilian alike—and we see the ravages of mom depletion every day. Clients and industry experts have long urged us to combine our wisdom to create a scientific and practical program that targets moms specifically. So this is just what we've done.

Ashley Koff, a registered dietitian and the founder of her own nutrition counseling and consulting company, brings smart nutrition ideas on turning energy zappers into energy sustainers to *Mom Energy*. Ashley was the expert dietitian behind *The Huffington Post Living*'s "Total Energy Makeover with Ashley Koff RD," the CW's *Shedding for the Wedding*, and Lifetime's *Love Handles*. She's also the resident dietitian for ESPN's newest outlet—espnW—and a contributing editor for *Natural Health* magazine.

Three years ago, Ashley launched Ashley Koff Approved (AKA)—a service to audit foods, supplements, and beauty products and the services that incorporate them to determine if they deliver on being part of a healthy lifestyle. To date, she has audited more than 10,000 products and services to decide whether or not they will get the coveted tagline "AKA can't be bought, it's earned." Obviously, Ashley knows a thing or two about energy.

Kathy, the other half of our team, has been a household name in the fitness and health industry for longer than she'd like to admit. Not only was she a regular fitness correspondent on the *Today* show for 13 years and an inductee in the National Fitness Hall of Fame, but she's also worked with stars such as Julia Roberts, Michelle Pfeiffer, Cindy Crawford, Jennifer Aniston, Drew Barrymore, Claudia Schiffer, Kim Basinger, and Angie Harmon—many of whom were excited to let us share their secrets in this book. Oh, and did we mention that Kathy's got three rambunctious school-aged boys (two of whom are teenage twins)? So as a full-time mom and a full-time trainer, Kathy continues to shape the bodies and inspire the lives of millions around the world. And in *Mom Energy*, she shares her energy-enhancing fitness secrets and teaches you how to easily fit healthy activity into your already busy lives.

So suffice it to say, we've been tireless crusaders of health and well-being for a long time, and now we're here to help you get the energy you want by giving you straightforward and effective energy-optimizing techniques that you don't normally find elsewhere. So no, there are no secrets. It's not magic. And we are not genies who will simply give you your three energy wishes. We are realists—practical Midwesterners at the core. We believe in basic and doable, but we also believe in effort.

ENERGY AND HEALTH

Vis viva is Latin for "living force"—it's that internal part of us that makes us feel alive and energetic. And it may be the ultimate marker of optimal health. Poor energy levels don't just mean that you won't get everything done; they are also warning signs that your health has declined, that your body's systems aren't operating at their best.

The body is an energetic force—it's dynamic and can be viewed as a collection of intricate energy equations (don't worry, there won't be any math). If one of those equations isn't balanced, the whole system starts to falter. Like a crack in a window that changes the climate of the entire house. One of the chief goals of this book is to help you understand how the core concepts of physiologic energy relate to your individual body and sense of well-being.

> Lack of energy is one of the top five complaints doctors hear from patients. Unfortunately,
> you can't buy energy, but once you learn how to achieve mom energy, it lasts forever.

And when you focus on balancing your energy equations and accelerating your energy levels naturally—as we will show you—everything else begins to fall into place. You'll lose unwanted weight. You'll boost your immune system and have fewer colds each year. You'll sleep like a baby at night. Your skin will glow and your wrinkles will go. You'll ignite your relationships (and sex life!). You'll enhance your productivity and ability to get things done. You'll know how to have that cake and eat it, too, without it sabotaging anything. You'll be able to manage stress better and cope with whatever life throws you (or takes away from you). You'll experience greater happiness and well-being. And you'll automatically find the motivation to keep moving forward with optimism and fortitude. We can't guarantee that we'll cure disease or make special health challenges go away, but we're pretty certain that if you can follow at least some of the guidelines and suggestions in this book, you'll start to notice a better you. You'll sense that sustained, good energy levels make previously difficult health issues weaker and less bothersome.

ENERGY FOR SALE

If you could put energy in a bottle, you'd be rich. Maybe that's why the "energy industry" is still booming despite the economy. PowerBar. Red Bull. Amp. Venom. Accelerade. Super Energizer. Energice. SoBe Adrenaline Rush. The number of drinks, herbs, bars, and even goo that sell energy continues to climb. Sales of these quick fixes have more than quadrupled in the last decade.

But even if you buy into this market, you know that caffeine and quick sugar fixes can only go so far to boost your energy in the short-term. These tactics can, in fact, trip a vicious cycle that spirals downward into the pits of total energy depletion. That's right: every time you pick up a can of soda or energy bar, you could be downshifting your body into reverse. Yes, these products do give you that initial jolt, but in doing so they can trigger a cascade that ends in energy exhaustion. In other words, most of those energy blasts are responsible for creating energy imbalances that result in feelings of being tired, worn, sapped, unwell, and, quite frankly, useless.

So if the energy industry can't sell us the cure for this energy crisis, what can we do? The answer: adopt lifestyle habits that naturally infuse you with energy. And that means coming to terms with the economics of your own energy equation so you can then manage it effectively. That's what *Mom Energy* is all about.

We've put together a three-part strategy that entails Reorganizing your time and eating patterns, Rehabilitating your physical body, and Recharging through attention to exercise, sleep, and play. We'll start the book, however, with some groundwork. In Part I ("Before You Get Started") we'll take you on a revealing tour of how our body's energy equations function to either keep us fully charged or leave us depleted; plus we'll offer a series of self-tests that you can take to gauge where you are on the energy spectrum, as well as determine your unique energy profile. This will set you up for embarking on your own personalized energy makeover in the remaining chapters, which are laid out in the order of your three-part strategy: Reorganize, Rehabilitate, and Recharge.

You'll know how to tailor specific goals to the suggestions detailed in Parts II through IV, and instigate slight shifts attuned to your lifestyle.

Because many of the chapters are chock-full of information and ideas, we've made it really simple by adding a section titled "Mom Up: Jump-Start Your Transformation" that gives you a simple and concrete takeaway to try and execute in your life that day or week. We understand that it can take time to implement all the strategies in this book. Sometimes, it helps to just start with one technique, one actionable step. So that's why we'll give you just that and avoid overwhelming you with too much to do. After all, you already have plenty on your plate!

Stop "Lifestyle Cycling"

We all fall into the trap of believing that there's a one-stop solution to the mom-energy problem. If we didn't believe in magic or "secrets" to looking and feeling great, then we wouldn't consume so much content from the magazines that shout out something new to try every month or, in some cases, every day. Admit it: you've heeded countless pieces of advice dispensed from a magazine, blog, or article to give yourself a boost. You manage to stick to a new regimen for a while, but then life—and that probably includes your kids—gets in the way of your efforts.

Over and over again we watch women cycle through one lifestyle trend to another, always ending back where they started and more energy-depleted.

So there must be (and there is) an alternative. You can learn how to stop cycling for good, to live a life that naturally infuses you with energy for the long term. It's about being the best that you can be. It's also about choosing where to put your efforts in the hopes of gaining some benefit in your health and well-being. By educating you to find your individual *vis viva,* we empower you to succeed via your own choices, not another's dogma.

Health is dynamic; energy is dynamic; the body is dynamic. Neither energy nor health is something you get to achieve and cross off your list like purchased groceries or an accomplished task. Just as becoming a mom means you're a mom forever, you'll also never be done with seeking optimal health. The intensity of it will ebb and flow throughout your life, but that's just life! So let's make the most of it.

HELP FOR ALL MOMS

Celebrities may have more money and get more attention, but that doesn't make them more innately energetic or able to feel as good as the public photos and interviews let on. Whether the call comes in for us to fine-tune an actress's diet and exercise routine or put her through a major overhaul, there's a common thread in their "cure": getting results means learning how to make the most effective and efficient choices for them and their families too. They still have to do the work, even though someone else may be footing the bill, and their job rarely allows them to sit there looking good. These ladies are on the move, so they need a total energy solution—not just a quick-fix diet and tone-up plan. They want to have the zip to get through a long day and not feel like a truck has run them over by the end of it.

Take Julia Roberts, for example. Before she was married with kids she filmed *America's Sweethearts* with Catherine Zeta-Jones in Las Vegas. It wasn't all that demanding of a role physically (it wasn't an action film filled with crazy stunts), but with any movie schedule you have to be on and ready at all times. So the days can go on and on, and there's a real need to have an underlying level of energy that you can draw from at any given time. Now Julia has entered another dimension with three kids and a husband, and you'll hear about some of her tricks in later chapters.

Another example is Michelle Pfeiffer. When she played Cat-woman in *Batman Returns*, she had to be up at 4 A.M. so she could get a workout in and be on the set by 6 A.M. The days would wear on into the evening past seven o'clock sometimes. This film did have a lot of action, and you'll recall Michelle donned a skin-tight catsuit. But for her the request was: "I need to be able to get through the day on little sleep; I'm up early and the shooting days are long and grueling. Help!"

Even if you're not on a set slugging out 16-hour days, you've got your own version of that grueling job. You've got your own set of shifts from being a mom to being a wife, a daughter, a sister, an employee or boss of your own company, a friend, and back to being a mom again, over and over again. Women today are redefining the workforce and changing all the rules. Now that 51 percent of the workforce is comprised of women—and the majority of those women are moms—it's time that they got their own personal guide.

We all can agree that moms shoulder a whole different set of challenges than our male counterparts. We don't know any mothers who aren't up at the crack of dawn and still awake long after they should have gone to bed. The time has come for them to get some serious attention and lifesaving tips attuned to their sense and sensibilities.

GET READY TO REV

The good news is becoming fully charged doesn't require a complete shift in your lifestyle or denying yourself things you really enjoy. And the best news is it doesn't have to cost more or take more time. This book is for all of us who have ever looked in the mirror and wished we could hit reboot.

PART I

BEFORE YOU GET STARTED

CHAPTER 1

Master Your Body's Native Energy Language

Women can have so much more than they realize.
I feel very lucky that I've had the opportunity to try to grasp as
much as I can in my life. So, I do have a family, and I do
have a husband, and I do have a career. And not at one time
do I feel that I'm 100 percent in any one [of them].
That means that every day it's a navigation . . .

— BROOKE SHIELDS

"I can't lose my belly fat. The words *vibrant* and *well rested* are no longer part of my vocabulary. Feeling stressed out and overstimulated is my life. Don't tell me to give up my caffeine, wine, bread, and sugar. I don't remember the last time I went on a diet that worked. They never work! I dream of looking and feeling younger, but have no idea how to without making unrealistic changes that ain't ever gonna happen. I hate being tired all the time. I hate feeling like road-kill. I don't remember the last time I felt sexy and desirable."

Do any of these statements sound familiar? You'd think the word *mom* stands for "Missing Our Mojo." Yet losing your mojo isn't what you signed up for, and it doesn't have to be your reality. Even if you're the most health conscious of moms, if you're like any of the people we counsel, you still find yourself blinking in disbelief and feeling wiped out in ways you never expected and can't rebound from. You can seemingly be doing everything "right" but still sputter on low ebb and low energy (unable to lose those last 10 to 20 pounds or fit into your skinny jeans without fasting for a month).

In this chapter, we're going to take you on a quick tour of your body's energy physiology, and help you begin to see where you might be going wrong, and where there's room for improvement.

THE PHYSIOLOGY OF ENERGY

The word *energy* is quite loaded these days, and you're probably more apt to think about energy in terms of oil or electricity than biology. But the physiology of energy is very real, and more tied into your health than anything else. In fact, if you picked up this book thinking you'd find better secrets to weight loss, or to sleep better, lower your risk for disease, and manage chronic conditions, then look no further than your own energy physiology to help you with all that and much more. It's a shame that we seem to focus so intently on one single area, such as stubborn belly fat or insomnia, when we can help all the important areas in our lives if we just focus on the dynamics of our body's energy. So we want to begin by asking the question: what does energy mean to you? More succinctly, what does energy imbalance mean to you?

When we asked a few fantastic moms to speak about the meaning of an "energy imbalance," we were delightfully surprised by some of the answers we got:

> Energy imbalance is one of the main causes for most of our health issues here in America. To me, energy imbalance means that people are not naturally creating or using energy throughout the day, which causes more exaggerated highs and lows of energy.

Energy imbalance could very well be the number one issue of our time. Most women wear far more hats than they should. Mothers often act as breadwinners, chefs, chauffeurs, the cleaning service, secretary, accountant, and, oh yes, family psychologist. All the while attempting to love herself, which is often the very last thing she has the time or energy for.

I feel better when the energy that I access in my work on a daily basis—i.e., my mind—is balanced by the energy that I access for exercise—my body. By balancing the two of them, I feel I can access the energy that nourishes my spirit.

Energy imbalance means a deficiency in one or more of the following: nutrition, exercise, sleep, and "me time." If any of these are not at an optimum level, it lowers my productivity, immune system, and positive family dynamics.

[E]nergy problems stem from a poor diet, lack of exercise, and allowing ourselves to be stretched too thin. As caregivers, we often forget to take care of ourselves.

Now that's a set of some seriously smart responses! But it's true: there's plenty of science to help explain how energy imbalance lies at the root of many health problems, which we'll get to shortly. Put simply, when you focus on optimizing your energy levels (naturally, not with stimulants that can temporarily give the illusion of energy), you support optimal health. Energy = Health. And when you have health, you have energy. In other words, you feel great.

THE ECONOMICS OF YOUR BODY'S ENERGY METABOLISM

Although every aspect of your life depends on energy, the concept of energy from a biological standpoint can be difficult to grasp. Energy, after all, cannot be seen or touched. It manifests in various forms, including thermal, mechanical, electrical, and chemical energy. And obviously we're not just talking about energy in terms of engineering and the universe at large à la Newtonian physics. It gets much simpler and down-to-earth than that! In the body, thermal energy helps us to maintain a constant body temperature, mechanical energy helps us to move, and electrical energy sends nerve impulses and fires signals to and from our brains. Energy is stored in foods and in the body as chemical energy.

The body is an energetic force—it's dynamic, and its operations can be viewed as a collection of basic, interlocking energy equations. Those equations are what make up our metabolism, which is the total sum of all the reactions that the body uses to obtain or expend energy from what we consume. If any one of those equations isn't fully functional, the whole system is impacted, and with sufficient disruption the system itself can start to falter. When that happens you can kiss being energized good-bye.

There is no better and no more reliable barometer of your overall health than your perceived energy level. Yep. Very low-tech but as accurate a diagnostic tool in determining general health as you'll find. If you're feeling low on energy, that's an extremely reliable indicator that there's a systemic health problem or issue that needs attending—your interlocking "equations" are not humming. That's why doctors recognize chronic exhaustion and low energy as a red flag signaling a potentially serious decline in health; it's a cue that the body's operations are falling apart. Persistent fatigue, for instance, is one of the most commonly experienced cancer symptoms. It's also usually the case that the more fatigue, the more advanced the cancer—both malignant and benign. Cancer is a prime example of a disease state whereby the body is not performing at 100 percent as it creates unhealthy cells that further disrupt other systems. The mere presence of cancer can increase your body's need for energy, weaken your muscles, and alter your hormones—all of which lead to fatigue. Needless to say, add any treatments like chemotherapy on top of that and you can see why cancer patients feel chronically tired. This isn't to say that being low on energy means you have cancer; we mention this link because it clearly illustrates—to the extreme—the association between true health and energy. And it points to the fact that taking control of your health (and so much more!) hinges on addressing energy levels.

Before moving forward, we want to be clear that "mom energy" is not about "high energy." It's unrealistic to think you won't ever have days when your energy is below average. Life happens, and energy can wane for a variety of reasons—not all of them necessarily bad. What we want to show you, however, is how to work toward having sustained energy and how to respond to inevitable fluctuations in your energy so you can avoid pitfalls and long-term consequences. You can also avoid putting yourself at a higher risk for disease and, yes, even ailments as serious as cancer. Also bear in mind that being low on energy or having an off day is not synonymous with a bad mood.

When it comes to this concept of having and actually feeling energy, we're not just talking about your perceived energy and sense of whether or not you can withstand walking a mile uphill today with your kids in tow. We're referring to a very real and critically important set of reactions and processes in the body that ultimately do determine how energetic you feel. And it all boils down to energy metabolism—the biochemical processes that occur within a living organism to maintain life.

Energy Metabolism 101

The science of metabolism is staggering, and we don't expect you to understand the biology in a way that a doctor or even your high-school science teacher would. It won't help you to maximize your energy, or your metabolism for that matter.

The nutrients in particular that the body breaks down into basic units are carbohydrates, fats, and proteins. From carbohydrates come glucose, your body's—especially the brain's—primary form of fuel; from fats we get glycerol and fatty acids, many of which are essential ingredients in hormones and the protective sheath in our brain that covers communicating neurons; and from proteins we get amino acids, which are the building blocks to lots of structures, including our blood, muscle, skin, organs, antibodies, hair, and fingernails.

Each of these nutrients travels down a different pathway, but all can eventually fuel the body's production of ATP (adenosine triphosphate), which is essentially our bodies' ultimate energy currency. ATP is a high-energy compound that fuels biochemical reactions in the cells. It's responsible for charging our metabolic engines, allowing our muscles to move and our brains to think, and supplying our enzymes with the energy they need to catalyze chemical reactions. ATP is produced continuously throughout the day using the energy from the breakdown of foods. Clearly, what you choose to eat will affect your body's production of ATP, and how you choose to move will also affect your body's use—and need for—adequate ATP. A mom who gets up before dawn to run five miles before the kids get up will have a radically different ATP-producing machine than a mom who sleeps in and has a pancake breakfast with her little ones. That said, each mom's different routine has its own mom-energy merits, and you'll soon come to understand the difference.

The energy-creating centers in our bodies are mitochondria—tiny organelles found inside all of your cells. Your mitochondria are probably the most important structures in your cells. Most cells in the human body contain somewhere between 500 and 2,000 mitochondria, and they make up as much as 60 percent of the volume of muscle cells. Not only do your mitochondria convert the stored energy in fat, protein, and carbohydrates into ATP, but they are involved in almost every energy-intensive process in the cell. Many diseases that deal with energy balances, from diabetes to muscle wasting as one ages, can be traced back to defects in a cell's mitochondria. In fact, mitochondria have their own DNA, so they don't have to depend on the nucleus to repair or replace themselves.

> Mitochondria convert calories and oxygen into energy the body can use: adenosine triphosphate (ATP). Your cells contain about 100,000 trillion mitochondria, which consume 90 percent of the oxygen you breathe. This oxygen is necessary to burn the calories we eat in food.

Your body's metabolism is constantly in motion, even as you sleep or sit on a couch zoned out while watching TV. The body will seek resources it needs from the raw materials you feed it. And when those raw materials run low, the body will work its magic to create its own source wherever possible. Case in point: Most cells can produce glycogen, which is a stored form of glucose. But the liver and muscle cells store the greatest amounts. After you eat, liver cells obtain the glucose from the blood and convert it to glycogen. Between meals, when blood glucose levels fall, the reaction is reversed, and glucose is released into the blood. This ensures that cells will have a continual supply of glucose to support life. When you take in more carbs than your body can store as glycogen or are needed for normal activities, all that extra glucose becomes fat and is then deposited into your fat cells. The body has an almost unlimited capacity to do this type of conversion, which is why chronic overeating usually leads to obesity.

CAUSE AND EFFECT

One of the easiest ways to understand the dynamics of the body is to consider what can happen when something gets out of whack, or when there is too much of one ingredient and not enough of another. This is true not just for moms, but for their brood as well. In 2009, reports emerged about a rise in kids getting kidney stones, which may seem unusual but not when you consider the huge amounts of processed foods that our kids are eating these days. Eating too much salt, coupled with not eating enough water-rich foods or drinking enough water to help counter that salt, can result in excess calcium in the urine, which sets up conditions for kidney stones to develop.

Johns Hopkins Children's Center in Baltimore, a referral center for children with kidney stones, used to treat one or two youngsters annually 15 or so years ago. Now it tracks new cases every week. Virtually all hospitals across the country have noticed an increase, puzzling some doctors but confirming to others the repercussions of a high-salt diet—even in children. Unfortunately, convenience foods marketed to kids and their busy parents (ahem!) are often high on the salt meter and low on the water meter. Some examples: chicken nuggets, finger foods such as little sausages and pickles, hot dogs, ramen noodles, canned spaghetti, packaged deli meats, and candy bars.

Whether the rise in kidney stones among kids can be wholly blamed on a salty diet is still up for debate. A metabolic problem also may be in play, but the message is clear: too much salt has a profound effect on the body at any age, and can exacerbate existing problems. You have probably heard about gallstones, which affect up to 20 million Americans and are twice as common among women. This is another example of what can happen when there's an imbalance in the body, as gallstone formation is thought to be due to an imbalance of bile salts and minerals, dehydration, toxins, and excess cholesterol in the bile. The condition is also associated with a high-fat, low-fiber diet and pregnancy. When the delicate ratio that keeps bile in liquid form is imbalanced, crystals ("stones") form from some of those bile components. They can be a real medical problem, blocking the flow of bile from the liver and gallbladder, and sometimes obstructing the pancreas and intestines as well.

Another case of biological cause-and-effect is found in the balance of calcium and magnesium. When we consume more calcium and not enough magnesium, the body notes this excess by failing to sufficiently relax when it should. Due to food processing and a lack of whole grains and legumes in the diet, we see a several-fold decline in magnesium while calcium intake from food and supplements stays steady, thus often resulting in a "conditional deficiency" of magnesium. Since magnesium turns off the body's stress response (inside the cells) and allows for muscle relaxation, this cause-and-effect relationship can cause a very stressful, tight, constipated effect from head to toe, most often affecting one's ability to fall and stay asleep.

We'll give you another example that most people can relate to: sleep. If you don't get enough sleep to keep your body's engine humming, you'll start to throw your appetite hormones out of whack. Sleep is not a luxury.

The two digestive hormones that control your feelings of hunger and appetite are ghrelin and leptin. As with many hormones, these two are paired together but have opposing functions. One says "go" and the other says "stop." Ghrelin (your "go" hormone) gets secreted by the stomach when it's empty and increases your appetite. It sends a message to your brain that you need to eat. When your stomach is full, fat cells usher out leptin (your "stop" hormone) so your brain gets the message that you are full and need to stop eating. A bad night's sleep—or just not enough sleep—creates an imbalance of both ghrelin and leptin. Studies now prove that when people are allowed just four hours of sleep a night for two nights, they experience a 20 percent drop in leptin and an increase in ghrelin. They also have a marked increase (about 24 percent) in hunger and appetite. And what do they gravitate toward? Calorie-dense, high-carbohydrate foods like sweets, salty snacks, and starchy foods. Sleep loss essentially disconnects your brain from your stomach, leading to mindless eating. It deceives your body into believing it's hungry (when it's not), and it also tricks you into craving foods that can sabotage a healthy diet.

Poor sleep catches up to most moms. It also sets moms up for entering a vicious cycle whereby they plunge into deeper sleep deprivation (and reel from its numerous negative effects), and avoid healthy behaviors that can counter the bad mood, such as exercise and eating right. So even if you say you're okay on four or five hours, you should take a good look at your sleep habits if you are unhappy with your energy, not to mention your looks and your weight. See what happens when you force yourself to get more sleep. You just might force yourself to lose unwanted weight and achieve a more beautiful, energetic you. We'll be going into much more detail about sleep in Chapter 9.

A THREE-DIMENSIONAL PICTURE

When thinking about how to simplify the complex mechanics of the human body's energy-manufacturing processes and the seemingly dazzling feats made by the body to sustain life, we thought it helpful to consider three unique dimensions to your overall energy equation. We'll take a quick look at each of these factors here and, throughout the book, come to see how all of these merge together to determine whether you're running on renewable sources of energy or perpetually struggling to find a charging station.

The First Dimension: Your Body's Composition

The three main components in your body are water, muscle, and fat. We're taking some liberties here—our bodies are much more complex than that—but let's focus for a moment on these three big components that do, in fact, contribute largely to the puzzle of our energetic lives.

Waterworks: If you were listening in high-school biology class, then you already know that we are watery creatures. Our bodies are about 75 percent water, so water is a huge factor in your energy, not to mention your survival. Water helps keep your overall metabolism and all other bodily processes functioning properly. Our body's water needs are so critical that if the water content in our blood drops below normal, muscle cells will leach water to support the flow necessary in the blood. When this happens, we become dehydrated. Diets that severely restrict carbohydrates may give people the illusion of sudden weight loss, but here's why: cutting off carbohydrates forces the body to find other sources of energy. It likely turns to glycogen, which is stored carbohydrates on reserve in your muscles and liver. Once glycogen storages are tapped, water gets released. So someone who cuts back on carbohydrates and notices sudden weight loss could be shedding just water weight rather than real fat weight. This could then prompt further dehydration and undeniable hunger.

There's another aspect to this water equation. Not only do fat cells need water to convert fat to usable forms of energy, but your muscles also need water to perform. So when you increase your physical activity, your muscles will store more glycogen with water to meet the demands you're placing on them. Likewise, your bloodstream will carry more water, upping the amount of blood traveling through your system to deliver much-needed oxygen to your muscles. All of this action means a higher level of energy efficiency and a bigger capacity to burn calories—and, in turn, burn fat. It's not a surprise that people who can burn fat easily are using energy more efficiently; as a result, they also feel more energetic as well. The proverbial couch potato will be less efficient and, subsequently, feel less energetic.

The Muscle Factor: People forget how valuable muscle mass is to quality of life, longevity, and the ability to maximize energy. Certainly genetics and special conditions, such as thyroid issues, can come into play, but the overriding factor in both weight gain and metabolic rate is muscle mass.

Unlike fat, muscle is a high-maintenance tissue. It's in constant use by the body, and as such it requires a lot of energy to keep it in good working order. This helps explain why lean, more muscular people have an easier time burning calories at rest than do people with higher proportions of body fat. Muscle burns calories, whereas fat just stores them. Calories, by the way, are units of energy. Your basal metabolic rate is the energy—measured in

Don't confuse "energy density" with food that
will infuse you with "high energy." In a nutshell,
energy density refers to the number of calories in
a particular volume or weight of food. High-energy-
density foods, such as an apple fritter, pack a lot
of calories per bite; conversely, low-energy-density
foods, such as a regular apple, contain fewer calories per bite. Bite for bite, or ounce for ounce,
you'll consume more calories—not all of which
will be necessary to sustain your body's needs
and keep your energy running on high. In other
words, high-energy-density foods can sabotage
your efforts to optimize your energy. Don't panic:
if this sounds confusing, you'll soon understand
what we're talking about. For now, bear in mind
that low-calorie foods (low-energy-density) that
can infuse you with real energy do exist. We'll be
showing you exactly that in Chapter 5.

calories—that your body needs daily for your cells to function
properly and to stay alive. It's what you burn without exerting any
effort. Most women need a daily average of 1,500 to 1,800 calories.
Of course, this depends on activity levels, body size, and body
type. To lose a pound of fat, you have to burn 3,500 more calories
than you consume. For example, if you cut back on calories and
increase your exercise so that you create a 500-calorie daily deficit,
you'd burn enough extra fat to lose a pound in a week.

We get asked all the time: isn't a calorie the same in all foods?
In theory, yes, but not when you consider how the body responds
to calories from different sources. A chocolate chip muffin, for
example, can be chock-full of calories coming from sugars that

will likely get stored in your fat cells. This happens due to the spike in insulin that occurs when you eat that tasty muffin. The insulin tells your body to store the extra—what the body doesn't need for immediate energy—as fat. Eating a deli sandwich on one slice of whole-grain bread with organic turkey, bell peppers, and avocado, on the other hand, won't cause the same surge in insulin and, in fact, requires time and an expenditure of energy to break down its proteins, healthy fats, and carbohydrates. The sandwich will keep your energy sustained and balanced.

> People who go to extremes to lose weight quickly often impair their fat metabolism by cutting too far back on calories, which forces the body into starvation mode. When this happens, the body holds on tightly to fat and burns up muscle tissue for energy—two counterproductive events to fat loss, energy conservation, and overall health.

People whose muscle-to-fat ratio is high feel more energized and motivated to stay active. And it's not just about the muscle fibers that allow us to move and exercise. Involuntary muscle activities are going on continuously to keep you alive. Your heart, which itself is a muscle, pumps oxygen and nutrients to cells; muscle action pumps lymph through your lymphatic system as part of your immune system; breathing depends on muscles to deliver oxygen; and muscle activity in the skin allows you to sweat and maintain your temperature.

Every year after age 25, our body's composition begins to shift quite dramatically. We gain, on average, about one pound of body weight each year and lose a third to a half pound of muscle. As a result, our resting metabolism decreases approximately 0.5 percent annually. So unless you downshift your caloric intake as your metabolism slows down, you'll experience frustrating weight gain, which can then inhibit optimal energy metabolism.

Although losing a fraction of muscle mass each year may seem minuscule, it adds up to be quite significant—translating to about a 1 to 2 percent loss of strength each year. With this loss of muscle strength, we tend to spontaneously become less active because daily activities become more difficult and exhausting to perform. We, in effect, lose energy more easily just like an old car that hasn't been serviced in a while will use up more gas than a new, efficient model.

Women have special challenges in the fat vs. muscle department. Because on average we don't have as much testosterone as men, it's harder for us to build and maintain muscle mass. This partly explains why recent research suggests that we'll lose muscle mass twice as fast as men of the same age. Add to that any hormonal challenges or conditions like diabetes and you can see why women have a harder time losing weight and keeping it off than men do.

In this book, we're going to challenge you to pay closer attention to your muscle mass than your fat mass. It's not that we wouldn't want you to lose excess fat, but when you put the focus on muscle—a positive, energy-grabbing tissue—then you will automatically tip the scales in favor of muscle and effortlessly gain more energy. And yes, this will include a bow to physical fitness as well as nutritional sense. *Fitness* is really a word that means fit to metabolize energy efficiently. When you're fit, you can create energy optimally. A fit person is an energetic person.

The Truth about Fat: In the past decade, scientists have uncovered a wealth of knowledge about types of body fat. Like cholesterol, there are good and bad types. Just last year researchers discovered an alarming difference between brown, or "good," fat and the more predominant "bad" fat, which tends to be white or yellow and collects around the waistline. Brown fat, which actually has a brownish tint to it, is stored mostly around the neck and under the collarbone (so, to a large extent, it's invisible). This fat encourages the body to burn calories to generate body heat (ahem: energy!), and plays an important role in keeping infants warm (infants, as we all know, have fatty necks). Until very recently we believed that this fat was either gone or no longer active by adulthood. Much to the contrary, it may have a huge role in our ability to stay lean as adults. These recent studies found that lean people have far more brown fat than overweight and obese people, especially among older folks. Unlike its bad-fat counterpart, brown fat burns far more calories and generates more body heat when people are in a cooler environment. Women are more likely to have it than men, and women's fat deposits are larger and more active.

The unhealthy fat that collects around the waistline is often referred to as visceral fat, because it collects around the "viscera"— your vital organs such as your heart, liver, and lungs. And it doesn't just sit there. Visceral fat is metabolically active, but instead of burning lots of calories, it prefers to release chemicals that affect your metabolism—negatively. Put simply, it can impact the balance of your body's interlocking equations. Excess calories stored as body fat generate hormones that can cause weight gain while preventing the production of healthy substances that can lead to weight loss. We are just beginning to understand how visceral fat can change the body's chemistry and work against any attempts to lose weight and fight disease—or to sustain energy, for that matter.

Visceral fat is an age maker and energy depleter—it wreaks havoc on the liver and has been linked to a slew of health problems, including heart disease, diabetes, some forms of cancer, and a cluster of risk factors called metabolic syndrome, which increases the chance of developing these diseases. It should come as no surprise that the more visceral fat you have, the lower the amount of energy your body can create. Visceral fat is not a problem just for overweight or obese people. You can be thin and still have visceral fat if you're not fit. Because visceral fat is the most dangerous kind of fat, doctors have grown more concerned about waist size than the number on the scale, which can be very deceiving. While abdominal fat is usually visible, visceral fat can be hidden deep inside an outwardly "thin" person. The same holds true for fat that can line blood vessels, restrict blood flow, and damage the cardiovascular system.

The Second Dimension: Hormones

Is there any mom who isn't familiar with the power of hormones? Since the time you hit puberty you've been under the spell of raging hormones at least once a month. And certainly anyone who's been through pregnancy and childbirth definitely has a love-hate relationship with these powerful chemicals.

Because everything in the body is connected, shifts in hormones through the years can have profound effects on the body's energy system. From a physiological standpoint, hormones help control how you feel, such as hungry, thirsty, tired, hot, cold, horny, and down in the dumps. They also command where we are on life's continuum, from our childless days to our postmenopausal years when our bodies try to thrive on a totally different concentration of hormones.

Briefly, hormones are simply chemical messengers that travel in the body's blood vessels to target areas where they have an intended effect. These chemical messages, which are tiny in volume, have many large and important jobs, such as regulating metabolism, growth and development, tissue function, and even your mood. The body's hormonal system includes the sex glands (testes in men, ovaries in women), the kidneys, pancreas, hypothalamus, pituitary, pineal, parathyroid, thyroid, and adrenal glands. There are many hormones in the body. In addition to estrogen, the most familiar ones include progesterone, cortisol, adrenaline, and androgens such as testosterone. Every organ has certain hormones, and many hormones have multiple functions that overlap. When all hormones are balanced, the body works as it should, organs function properly, tissues are supple and resilient, and your energy-packing metabolism runs smoothly. Conversely, the smallest variation in hormone levels can cause great, sometimes catastrophic effects all over the body, including the systems that generate energy and make you feel energetic.

Exactly how our hormones ebb and flow quite automatically within us can take up a whole semester in biochemistry. In brief, when stress hits, cortisol tells our brains that we are hungry, so we then seek out food. "Stress," by the way, doesn't have to be the kind we experience while traversing a highway to make our exit. Eating a box of chocolates or a pint of premium ice cream when you're sad, frustrated, angry, and moody—all of which the body can interpret as being stressed—has its reasoning. Fatigue born out of sleep deprivation and a caffeine addiction also causes the body to cry out for energy. These cries come first for carbohydrates, the body's preferred source of energy, thanks to cortisol's message to our brain that demands sugary, fatty foods—all the wrong foods for stopping the cycle. Rich, sugary foods don't do much for us but contribute to insulin swings, poor blood-sugar balance, as well as extra pounds, potbellies, worse moods . . . and do we need to mention low energy?

What's more, the usual culprits—chips, cookies, quesadillas, bread and butter, my kid's ice cream—register in our brain's reward center in ways that make us crave them even more. When we give in, what we ingest dictates how the body will respond from there. We usually (1) don't choose well, and (2) overconsume when we are seeking carbs for energy. If we choose a sugary carb with fat, the combo can actually override our brain's satiety mechanism and we will keep eating (think ice cream, chips and guacamole, or cupcakes with icing). If we overconsume carbs, we get more energy than the body can use, and two things happen: (1) the extra gets stored as fat, and (2) we have more energy which then keeps us awake (if we are eating at night) or sets us up for another energy drop (what goes up must come down). This is what we call the carb hangover.

Another way to think of this cycle of carbohydrate overload is to consider each serving as a building block. When we have more than one block or have one without the balancing effect of other necessary blocks (ahem: healthy fats and proteins), then while our energy rises it also crashes. Some people may even get shaky due to hypoglycemia or other health conditions, or as a result of drinking caffeine at the same time. As you begin to worry about being able to function on low energy and fatigue sets in, the body will call out for sugar (that is, carbs) for energy. If you give in to this demand, which is primal, you'll awaken the body but create yet another vicious cycle—especially if you choose a low-quality form of carbohydrate. As we saw earlier, an imbalance of appetite hormones brought on by sleep deprivation alone can trigger an intense craving for foods high in fat, salt, and sugar. Recent research on the brain shows just how lethal this mix can be on the body, encouraging what's called conditioned hypereating, which short-circuits the body's self-regulating mechanisms, leading to chronic body chaos and energy loss.

We can tell ourselves that we're tired and acknowledge a deep hunger for "cheap" carbs, but then telling ourselves to avoid them can be extremely hard to do, if not impossible. Unfortunately, many of us remember feeling moody, low energy, or just darn deprived from the low- and no-carb diets that may have even worked, albeit temporarily. It isn't about carbohydrate avoidance; it's about learning to balance them, along with portion control and choosing better quality. While this may seem daunting or not like a "program" at all, it is indeed the energy solution that allows you to sustain energy and manage highs and lows that occur when life inevitably happens.

There's also new evidence to show that ingredients in some foods can disrupt your metabolism and your hormonal system, which impacts how well your body processes and burns energy. A class of natural and synthetic chemicals known as endocrine-disrupting chemicals (EDCs), also gaining the name "obesogens," can act in a variety of ways to make and keep you fat: by mimicking human hormones such as estrogen, by misprogramming stem cells to become fat cells, and, researchers think, by altering the function of genes. They enter our bodies through a variety of ways: from natural hormones found in foods, from hormones administered to animals, from plastics in some food and beverage packaging, from ingredients added to processed foods, and from pesticides sprayed on produce. The lesson: when you eat organic whole foods, your body recognizes them and you help stoke your body's metabolism. Translation: fat loss, sustained energy. (We'll be going into more details on this topic later.)

Suffice it to say that the amount of stress your body endures, both physical and psychological, profoundly affects your energy level. In Chapter 10 we'll share nuggets of wisdom about managing stress. We'll also reiterate throughout the book ways in which you can calm the storm of certain stress hormones that work against every effort to sustain energy—and health.

The hormones that control our blood chemistry stability, and insulin in particular, deserve our attention. We already mentioned insulin briefly, but later on we'll look deeper into how insulin commands so much of our energy metabolism. So many moms today, for example, try to operate with insulin resistance, a condition in which the cells become ineffective at using energy efficiently. Which brings us to the third dimension to the overall energy equation.

The Third Dimension: Health Conditions

In Chapter 6, we're going to give you the scoop on health conditions that could be undermining any efforts to gain better energy. From thyroid issues to anemia and plain old digestive disorders like constipation and irritable bowel, the state of your health in every system of your body will dictate the state of your energy level. As we've been covering, when there's a bleep in an organ, tissue, system, or group of cells, there's a misfire that culminates in an inefficient metabolism. Just one minor deficiency or miscue happening in the body can trigger a cascade of troubles that results in energy depletion. Conversely, it's hard, in fact, to be low on energy if your body is operating efficiently and there are no hidden health challenges. It's simple: if you don't give the body the excuse to downshift, it won't. But when there's a health issue to address and the body needs to fight a germ or make up for a dysfunction somewhere in the whole system, then you will certainly feel it. Your energy will be limited as your body uses all it can to heal, protect, and consolidate its resources, so the ones that are required to keep you alive are still available no matter what. The body doesn't necessarily care, for instance, that you feel energetic. It just wants to maintain its non-negotiable systems of survival such as your heart and lungs.

One condition in particular that you've no doubt heard about is called inflammation, and it has everything to do with energy. Inflammation is the common denominator to virtually all medical conditions. At this writing, a Google search on inflammation turns up about 114.8 million hits—and there will be many more by the time this book is in your hands. It's practically a celebrity on its own. We're all familiar with the kind of inflammation that accompanies cuts and bruises on our skin—that pain, swelling, and redness that emerges. If you suffer from allergies or arthritis you're also tuned in to what inflammation feels like. But inflammation goes much deeper than that and can happen in your organs and systems without you even knowing it—without you really feeling it per se.

Although inflammation is part of our bodies' natural defense mechanisms against foreign invaders such as bad bacteria, viruses, and toxins, too much inflammation can be harmful. When inflammation runs rampant or goes awry it can disrupt your immune system and lead to chronic problems and/or disease. It's like having your furnace turned on to keep you warm and comfortable; if that furnace doesn't turn off once a certain temperature is reached, then your environment is going to get hot, uncomfortable, and dangerous. Soon enough, things in that environment will start to become adversely affected.

Inflammation may not seem remotely related to energy but, in fact, volumes of international research prove just how insidious chronic inflammation can be on the body. Researchers are now discovering bridges between certain kinds of inflammation and our most pernicious degenerative diseases today, including heart disease, Alzheimer's disease, cancer, autoimmune diseases, diabetes, and accelerated aging in general. Virtually all chronic conditions have been linked to inflammation, which, put simply, creates an imbalance in your body that stimulates negative effects on your health and, as such, your energy.

At the center of inflammation is the concept of oxidative stress—"rusting," if you will, of your organs and tissues. This can happen both on the outside, causing wrinkles and premature aging, and on the inside where it can stiffen our blood vessels, damage cell membranes, and essentially wreak havoc. Oxidation happens everywhere in nature and is a normal part of our biology; it occurs during the natural process of metabolism, which again is simply the body's means of turning calories (energy) from food and oxygen from the air into energy usable by the body. Oxidation, then, is very much a part of our being, but when it begins to run amok or there's too much oxidation without a balance of antioxidant action, it can become harmful. "Oxidation," of course, entails oxygen, but not the kind we breathe. The form of oxygen that's the culprit here is simply "O" because it's not paired with another oxygen molecule (O_2).

Think of oxidation as a combustion process, and the exhaust is made up of by-products called free radicals that need to be controlled. A biologist at UC Berkeley estimates that free radicals damage the DNA inside one of our cells some 10,000 times a day.

You've also no doubt heard about free radicals by now. These are molecules that have lost an electron. Normally electrons spin around in pairs, but forces such as stress, pollution, ultraviolet light from the sun, and ordinary body activities (even breathing) can make one of them break off. When that happens, the molecule loses all sense of propriety and starts ricocheting around, trying to steal electrons from other molecules. This commotion is the oxidation process itself, a chain of events that attacks cells and kicks off inflammation, which creates more free radicals. Because oxidized tissues and cells don't function normally, the whole destructive process sets you up for a bevy of health challenges, from saggy skin and a low metabolism to obesity, heart disease, cancer, dementia, and other diseases. And as we've been covering, all of these resulting effects equate with low energy as the body is trying to constantly heal itself and repair DNA damage. It's no wonder that people with high levels of oxidation have an extensive list of symptoms: fatigue, brain fog, low resistance to infection, muscle weakness, joint pain, anxiety, headaches, depression, irritability, allergies . . . the list goes on and on.

As you can imagine, anything that reduces oxidation reduces the bad, chronic types of inflammation, and anything that reduces harmful inflammation reduces oxidation. That's partly why antioxidants are so important. These unselfish nutrients (including vitamins C, A, and E) donate electrons to free radicals, which interrupts the chain reaction and helps prevent the damage free radicals do. Historically, we ate food rich in antioxidants, such as plants, berries, and nuts. In the last century, the advent of advanced food manufacturing has radically changed how we eat. In the early 1900s, the processing and packaging of foods became an enormous growth industry; today, it's the largest industry in the world. Unfortunately, it's an industry that processes a lot of nutrients out of our diets that are sorely needed for optimal health and energy metabolism. Our bodies are equipped with their own antioxidants to protect us, but they are easily overwhelmed by poor diet.

While a detailed discussion of inflammation is beyond the scope of this book, we want you to keep in mind that the lifestyle you choose dictates the extent to which you experience inflammation. What you choose to eat for nourishment, for example, factors into this equation as much as the level of toxins you're exposed to or how much you engage in physical activity and reduce your stress. Foods high in processed sugars and unhealthy fats, for instance, can exacerbate inflammation. This, in turn, antagonizes energy metabolism and puts you at a higher risk for weight gain among a host of other health problems. It also sets in motion a vicious cycle that leads to more and more inflammation. The strategies in this book will point you in a direction toward the things you should be doing to support the natural structure and functions of your body so it maintains a healthy balance, limits inflammation, and ushers in optimal energy.

S P E A K I N G   Y O U R   B O D Y ' S   L A N G U A G E

Now that you have a general idea about how the body makes and uses energy, you can better understand the steps that need to be taken to balance your energy equation. You now speak the language of your body, which puts you way ahead of the game in the quest for energy.

The way most people think about "healthy eating" and "healthy lifestyle," based on the popular theories and headlines, is exactly the opposite of how our bodies actually work—and specifically how the body reacts and interacts with what we put in it and the environment around it. Topping the charts is our continuing obsession with counting calories, prioritizing carbs vs. protein vs. fat, and silly, overgeneralized nutritional recommendations for every body (one size fits all never works, especially when it comes to nutrition!). The diet business is a multibillion-dollar industry but the bottom line is: what it dishes out doesn't work.

Nevertheless, millions of people remain desperate to get healthy, feel energetic, and lose excess pounds, so they rededicate themselves to the same old strategies but will be doomed once more to disappointment in the long run. It is a telling benchmark of where things are that we devour advice that counsels healthy eating by swapping out your daily Whopper with cheese for a Big Mac. We can and must do better than that! But we often don't, or we think we're doing something right when it's actually a giant misstep that leads us in the wrong direction.

So, what do people use to live healthfully and feel energetic? We often hear about the tendency to have coffee in the morning, an energy bar in the afternoon, and a drink (or two) after work. In between these planned "energy boosts" there's the consumption of foods that must be unwrapped and which contain long lists of ingredients; and perhaps there's also a "master cleanse" once a year to clear everything out (and maybe drop a few pounds). The people who live like this believe they're doing the right thing. They're not eating huge meals or taking in excessive calories, and they believe their annual detox is sufficient. But are they really making the grade? Unfortunately, we think not.

As we mentioned before, sales of quick fixes—from ubiquitous energy bars and "health" drinks to odd-sounding powders, pills, extracts, and elixirs lining the aisles at popular health-food stores—have more than quadrupled in the last decade. The number of foods and beverages sold in packages with "natural" ingredients promising to do wondrous things to your health and longevity also has skyrocketed. In fact, as we write this, the makers of a popular drink, advertised as an antiaging dream-come-true that can lead to a "30 percent decrease in arterial plaque" and "17 percent improved blood flow," is being sued by the Federal Trade Commission for making false and unsubstantiated claims. Food health claims abound, and until the government clamps down on ads that tout specific health benefits, we must do a lot of the decoding ourselves. Even though on some level we want the pill or drink that does miracles, especially after experiencing the miracle of creating life, we know that life is more complex, and it's a gift—one that shouldn't be sold for $9.95 at a superstore or on QVC.

Despite what marketers would have you believe, there isn't one pill or drink that will work miracles. Yes, they do give you that jolt and the perception that they are doing something good for you, but here's the surprising truth: most of those energy blasts are responsible for creating energy imbalances! How does that happen?

To better understand this, let's look at body balance related to something all of us mothers remember: pregnancy. When you are pregnant, the body goes into a special mode to develop and protect the growing fetus. It gives the fetus total priority! Your immune system, for example, ticks down a notch to prevent your body from attacking your wondrous creation. And if your baby doesn't get the nutrients he or she needs in the womb, it will borrow from you IOU style—only it doesn't send a reminder for you to restock your stores. The reason you need extra calcium during pregnancy, for instance, is because your baby will take all the calcium from you and your food that it needs to grow. Any deficiencies you experience during pregnancy are more likely to harm the "host"—you!—over the long term. This type of exchange depletes energy reserves during pregnancy, which can affect your system all the way through grandmotherhood and beyond. The body will make sure there is calcium in the blood without worrying about taking it from the bone.

Caffeine, which is arguably the most commonly used (and abused) form of an energy blast, works in much the same way. While it may appear to aid or enable energy on some level, it throws energy off on other levels. Your heart, for instance, will tick a little faster in response to the caffeine, your liver will work a little harder to process the caffeine, and your kidneys will filter more fluid due to caffeine's diuretic effect. It's well documented that caffeine enhances performance, so you'll likely work a little harder and burn more energy while under the influence of caffeine, which can result in energy depletion, sleep deprivation, and perhaps a caffeine withdrawal headache once it's all gone. You've essentially robbed your long-term energy stores to get a short-term jolt, and the energy debt will be felt as low mood, exhaustion, and yes . . . less energy!

Don't get us wrong: there can be a time and place for caffeine, but you need to be aware of its hidden consequences. And as we'll see in Part II, the same can be said for other energy Band-Aids that offer an artificial boost.

Keep in mind that there is no single approach to optimizing energy, and neither diet nor exercise alone will balance your body's massive and complex energy equation. As this book clearly highlights, the combination of various habits, from how you stock your kitchen to how you manage stress, achieve restful sleep, cope with chronic conditions, and schedule exercise, are just a few of the important players in your energy level. Without a doubt, they also play into your health, happiness, and looks as well. It would be impossible to say which of these factors is more important. They all bear weight, and perhaps which one carries the most depends on your uniqueness, especially as they relate to your genetics and other lifestyle choices.

The Kickback Effect: energy can neither be created nor destroyed. That's basic physics. It helps to think of the body in these simple terms as well. When we burn lots of energy, we ask our bodies to work harder at creating more sources of energy.

Something else to keep in mind: we don't want to put too much energy in reserve (i.e., fat cells), because the body doesn't efficiently go to those cells when it needs energy. Instead, it calls out for more "new" energy, triggering that hankering for carbs, and typically low-quality carbs at that. It's like when your kids have plenty of school supplies, clothes, and toys but they still cry out for new ones.

CHAPTER 2

Determine Your Profile:
Put Your Energy
to the Test

The face you have at age 25
is the face God gave you,
but the face you have after 50
is the face you earned.

— CINDY CRAWFORD,
channeling Coco Chanel

It helps to have a general idea of where your overall energy stands today so you can maximize your journey forward and identify where you could be paying closer attention. This chapter presents two distinct tests. First you're going to find out how severe your energy lack is from a general standpoint, and then we'll help you identify which profile you fit so you can then customize the recommendations in this book to your life.

Quiz #1: How Low Is It?

Following is a brief quiz we've put together to help you gauge your level of energy—from the inside out. It's unlike other typical tests in the health category that you may have taken because we won't ask about your cholesterol level or number on the scale. Be honest with yourself as you answer these questions. You don't have to share your responses with anyone. We encourage you to revisit this quiz whenever you want, to see if any of your answers have changed for the better. You can always come back to this quiz as a way of checking in with yourself and see how you're doing.

1) I have caffeine (e.g., soda, coffee, tea, energy drinks):

   a. Never

   b. Only in the morning, to get me going

   c. Throughout the day; I should own stock in Coke

2) At 7 P.M. I feel:

   a. Hungry and tired

   b. Depressed

   c. Relaxed

3) I feel refreshed when I wake up in the morning:

   a. Most days

   b. Rarely, perhaps when on vacation

   c. Never—you've got to be joking

4) One glass of wine makes me:

   a. Chatty and relaxed in a good way

   b. Hungry and apt to indulge in high-carb or fatty foods

   c. Sleepy and oftentimes grumpy

5) I experience digestive issues (e.g., gas, bloating, constipation, acid reflux/heartburn, and/or diarrhea):

    a. Once a month, if that

    b. Once a week or more; check out my medicine cabinet

    c. Once in a blue moon

6) I crave sweets:

    a. Daily, usually midafternoon or at night

    b. When I'm stressed or during my period

    c. Rarely—I don't have a sweet tooth

7) I've been on a diet:

    a. Never

    b. Within the last year

    c. Since I was a teenager

8) The last time I initiated sex was:

    a. Last week—it was great

    b. Last year, I think

    c. I can't remember—who has the energy for that?

9) I can walk a mile in less than 14 minutes:

    a. Yes, I'm in great shape

    b. Are you kidding me? No, and I wish exercise weren't so important

    c. I have no clue

10) My kids and family typically:

a. Come first and I schedule time for myself around their schedule(s)

b. Adjust to my needs when I take time for myself

c. Never let me take a break; I can't even seem to put my foot down and schedule more time for myself

11) My sleep life is:

a. Dreamy: I love my sleep and get lots of it

b. So-so: Sometimes I sleep well, other times I don't

c. A nightmare: I rely on sleep aids frequently

12) My co-worker or friend would describe my energy as:

a. Nonexistent: I don't have a pulse

b. Hot and cold: I experience highs and lows

c. Pretty good: My energy is mostly consistent throughout the day

Answer yes or no to the following questions:

13) I buy products (e.g., bars, drinks, supplements) that promote their "energy" value.

Yes/No

14) I suffer from anxiety, restlessness, and/or depression (not necessarily diagnosed by my doctor).

Yes/No

15) I have an immediate family member who has one or more metabolic disease(s) or symptom(s): high blood sugar, high cholesterol, high waist circumference, high blood pressure, etc.

Yes/No

Scoring:

1. a (3 points); b (1 point); c (0 points)

2. a (1 point); b (0 points); c (3 points)

3. a (3 points); b (1 point); c (0 points)

4. a (3 points); b (1 point); c (0 points)

5. a (2 points); b (0 points); c (3 points)

6. a (0 points); b (2 points); c (3 points)

7. a (1 point); b (0 points); c (1 point)

8. a (3 points); b (1 point); c (0 points)

9. a (3 points); b (1 point); c (0 points)

10. a (0 points); b (3 points); c (1 point)

11. a (3 points); b (2 points); c (0 points)

12. a (0 points); b (1 point); c (3 points)

13. yes (1 points); no (3 points)

14. yes (0 points); no (3 points)

15. yes (0 points); no (3 points)

The lower your score, the less energy you have. Conversely, the higher your score, the more energy you have in your life.

If you scored below 10 points: You're barely holding on, and you know that you are laying the groundwork for some serious health consequences, too. You don't feel in control of your world, and you're never on your own priority list. The thought of exercising more, eating better, and focusing more on yourself sounds daunting and downright energy draining. The word *energy* makes you look around as if it's something you can buy (case in point: you bought this book!). We're guessing you hide the extent of the chaos pretty well from friends and family, but you know that if you don't get a handle on things soon, you're going to crack. *Energetic* is not a word you use very often.

You can't remember the last time you felt youthful and truly happy. You don't know what's good for you anymore because you've gotten so lost. And the dread of living like this for another year, let alone another day, is practically unbearable.

You have work to do and you know it, but the good news is one little step can result in a giant leap forward. We're here to help you catch your breath. It may take you time initially to get used to living by a new set of strategies and from a new perspective; but through the ideas presented in this book, you'll be able to shift how you live your life and learn to never let living low on energy steal your well-being again.

If you scored between 11 and 20 points: Your life needs a makeover, too, but you've seemingly got a better grip on things. You know you need to take action today or risk falling much further down the hole. You do try hard to keep all the balls in the air, but your juggling often leaves you exhausted emotionally and physically. The fatigue still lingers, the stress still accumulates like fat around your waist, and the mind still wanders down depressive paths when there's finally time. More than likely, energy highs and lows are a constant in your life because you reach for quick fixes and proverbial Band-Aids all the time. Despite knowing what's good for you deep down, you still struggle with gaining control over what's important in your life, and avoiding or limiting the things that you know bring your energy levels down. You have good, energetic days and you have days when your energy is so low you want to send your kids to someone else's house so you don't have to deal with them. Other people can easily suck your energy reserves, and you've never gotten good at saying no. And when it comes to your kids, they rule. But you're aware of this, which is why a little bit more effort and focus can propel you to where you really want to be: happier and more energetic every day.

If you scored above 20 points: You get the gold star. You're lucky to be part of a small but growing group of moms who work hard at maintaining balance in your lives with plenty of energy on reserve for those unexpected moments that require more out of you. But that work requires constant vigilance and attention. You know how easy it can be to slip up and then have to pay the consequences—physically, mentally, emotionally, and even spiritually. You still have moments of feeling guilty for taking time for yourself, or not being there for your children (or others in general) due to work, but you sense that your priorities are in some semblance of order because you don't feel that bad about yourself and your life. For you, this book will be a welcome reminder, and its fresh tips can help you to further fine-tune the good habits that keep you balanced and energetic on all levels.

> The ultimate question: If there was a pill for
> Mom Energy, but to get it you would have to do
> one of the following, which would you choose?
> (1) give up your child(ren) for six months; (2) break
> up with your partner; (3) move to an island with a
> book, a lover, and your favorite foods but no com-
> munication with the outside world; (4) run a Mom
> Energy weekly support group in addition to your
> current commitments; or (5) none of the above,
> I'd pass on the pill and deal with less energy.

QUIZ #2: IDENTIFY YOUR PROFILE: WHAT IS YOUR #1 ENERGY THIEF?

Now, let's see what type of energy makeover you need. The quiz below will help you to tailor the strategies in this book to your unique profile. We'll give you the focal points you need to maximize your journey forward.

We have found that there are typically five types of moms dealing with different challenges, and you can certainly have characteristics of more than one. Below are five checkboxes, each with questions that will help you to pinpoint your energy profile. Don't worry about checking more than one box, but see if you can relate to one of these profiles more so than the others. This mini quiz will identify your biggest issues and help you to personalize the ideas in this book to your life. Following the quiz are recommendations specific to each profile. You can read through them all if you like, and get out a highlighter and mark anything that resonates with you. Then, as you begin to make slight shifts in what you do each day, pay particular attention to what you highlighted and the suggestions specific to your profile.

Once you finish the quiz, make sure to remember which profile you identify with. While all parts of this book are helpful to all moms, there are some passages that will benefit people who fall in specific profiles more. As you're reading through, keep your eye out for the profile alert boxes that will draw your attention to specific sections. If your profile is listed in the profile alert, be sure to read those pages extra carefully. They should offer you specific solutions to your unique challenges.

❑   Do you suffer from a chronic condition such as irritable bowel, migraines, diabetes, fibromyalgia, depression, low thyroid, or any other medical conditions that have you taking (or contemplating) medication? Do you get sick a lot? Are you going through perimenopause or menopause?

»   If you answered Yes, then Profile 1 is for you.

❑   Would you consider yourself an insomniac? Do you have trouble falling asleep and staying asleep? Do you wake up feeling as if you never slept?

»   If you answered Yes, then Profile 2 is for you.

❑   Do you burn the candle at both ends? Are you

overloaded with To Dos, either at work, at home, or both? Would you consider yourself an emotional wreck?

» If you answered Yes, then Profile 3 is for you.

❑ Are you trying to lose weight? Have you been on a diet in the last year in an attempt to drop a few pounds? Are you on a diet now?

» If you answered Yes, then Profile 4 is for you.

❑ Do you feel stuck in a bad rut? Did you pick up this book because you feel as if you're struggling with every problem under the sun and need to break a vicious cycle of unhealthy habits that robs your energy . . . but you don't know where to start?

» If you answered Yes, then Profile 5 is for you.

Profile 1: The Medicine Cabinet

You may not have a medical diagnosis, but you do find yourself seeking relief from countless over-the-counter medications to keep up with chronic symptoms. It may be a lingering headache or a full-blown migraine. It may be an upset stomach or diarrhea. It may be premenstrual syndrome, perimenopause, or hot flashes from the real thing. It may be another backache (from playing with your toddler), or just a bad day working through a flare-up from your arthritis, fibromyalgia, or raging hormones. Suffering from a chronic condition leaves most people low or limited on energy. You feel awful with good reason, and your body chemistry isn't helping, especially if it's having to fight an illness, a shift in hormones, or just a passing cold.

Focal Points: Getting to the bottom of health conditions that could be affecting your energy is a must. Then, seeking proper treatment to help manage or, in some cases, cure your condition is also a must. Sometimes, however, treatments can entail medications that go against your energy reserves. In Chapter 6 we'll give you the information you need to make sense of some underlying medical aspects to energy—and energy depletion. This will help you to have the right conversation with your doctor. You may not, however, have to resort to drugs in all cases. It may just be that you need to focus on a few lifestyle changes to transform your health status and kick your condition to the curb. We can't promise any miracles here, but we've seen plenty of people change their health for the better and experience a surge in energy like never before, and which helps them to further manage or live with any irreversible condition.

Profile 2: The Mom Zombie

We get nearly an hour less sleep a day than we did 40 years ago. Juggling work and family seems to be the primary sleep thief. Medical conditions may also be at play. If you're going through menopause or are close to it, night sweats could be waking you up repeatedly. Or you could be lacking sleep due to the realities of a newborn baby, staying up to ensure your teenager makes it home safely, or paying bills late at night because 24 hours just isn't enough time. Or perhaps you can't turn off your mind to welcome sleep. And if you do, in fact, log a decent amount of sleep but it's not restful, then you could be suffering from a sleep disorder such as sleep apnea (which is actually quite treatable!). Whatever the cause, you've got a sleep deficit that's outstripped the national debt. And worrying about being tired adds to your anxiety and energy drain.

Given the problems we have with sleep lately, it's no wonder so many moms roam around like the walking dead during the day, alternating endless cups of coffee with cans of soda.

It's fine to consume caffeine in reasonable amounts (hey, it does serve a purpose and can deliver some beautifying antioxidants), but if you start living off the stuff, it can perpetuate an endless—sleepless—cycle that results in total energy depletion.

Focal Points: For you, getting a handle on your sleep will be your top priority (Chapter 9). This will likely entail rethinking your schedule and budgeting your time better (Chapter 3), how much caffeine you drink, and whether or not you really need to own stock in Starbucks. It's amazing how much one small shift, such as getting a good night's sleep on a consistent basis, can do to your overall health and energy levels. You might find, for example, that becoming a sound sleeper helps solve so many other challenges you've faced and makes it easier to deal with the kinds of adversity a mother encounters.

Profile 3: The Overworked and Overscheduled (and Overtired)

Moms who fit this profile are trying to do too much day and night. You can't seem to wean yourself from work—or your kids—enough to take any time for yourself. You might think that watching television late at night once the house is quiet with a tub of ice cream and/or a glass of wine is relaxing, but your body might be crying anything but. You're ripe for burnout, but the adrenaline that constantly fires through you somehow keeps you going. Deep down, though, you're probably suffering from some serious stress that could be sabotaging your health, from weight-loss goals to even your risk for things such as heart disease and cancer. Any energy you have is mostly fictitious—conjured by coffees and Cokes all day long.

Focal Points: Mom, you need to restructure your life! For you, getting a handle on your priorities and bringing your life—and your body—a semblance of balance will be key. Don't skip Chapter 3. No, you cannot do it all, but you can learn what your body needs most and how to provide for its optimal wellness. Even if you sleep pretty well, you probably burn through a lot of extra energy during the day unnecessarily. When you learn how to allocate your time and energy better, you won't crash into bed every night feeling like roadkill.

Profile 4: The Chronic Dieter

Chronic dieters are chronically energy depleted. In brief: traditional dieting typically revolves around restrictions and deprivations. Rather than a constant flow of energy, you experience highs and lows. And when you can't stand avoiding sugar any longer, you eat an entire box of cookies, sending your body's innate energy equations into a biological tailspin. Chronic dieters rarely make good examples for their children, either. You likely find yourself talking about weight ("I'm so fat!") in front of your kids without realizing it, and without knowing what that could be doing to their own sense of self and body-image issues.

Focal Points: If you're on a diet right now, stop! See if you can incorporate the strategies in this book without feeling as if you're on a traditional diet. You would do well to pay attention to all the chapters in this book, but pay closer attention to the nutritional aspects, especially Part II, which covers ideas on managing what you consume. Make it a goal to stop searching for hard and fast rules to what you should and shouldn't do, and instead, learn what you need as well as how to make the right choices for *you*. We won't demonize sugar, or any foods for that matter, but we will teach you how to enjoy all foods responsibly so none inflicts too much energy-depleting harm.

Profile 5: The Dead Battery

You go through the motions every day, clawing at every tip you read to feel better—and better about yourself—but nothing has worked. Maybe you're going through a divorce, or you've remarried and become a blended family with stubborn stepkids, or you have a capricious, explosive boss. . . . Whatever is going on, your energy (and confidence and self-esteem) has plummeted to the point that everyday irritants you'd normally blow off are getting to you at an alarming rate. Conversations with loved ones turn into arguments. You still say yes to too much, and harbor lots of resentment for doing so. Your diet is dead. Your attempts to exercise are dead. The person you thought you'd be as an amazing mom is dead. The only thing keeping you going is a big flood of stress hormones, but even that is not enough to recharge your battery.

Focal Points: For you, everything in this book will be helpful. Taking baby steps will be key so you don't give up entirely. Choose just one thing to do differently this week, then choose something else next week. Don't try to incorporate too many changes all at once. Take it slow. Rather than beat yourself up over "bad" habits, focus on creating new habits so there's no more room for the old ones. Focus on getting charged one day at a time versus being fully charged today with Band-Aid solutions. By learning which behaviors are the biggest energy detractors and how to exchange them for energy-gaining solutions, you will get charged and stay that way.

Most of us fit into one or more of these five mom profiles. As moms, we all get stuck in similar ruts at various times in our lives, and recognizing them for what they are makes it easier to combat them. Remember your profile and focal points because these will help you to maximize the ideas in the book for optimal results.

PART II

REORGANIZE

CHAPTER 3

Time Warp:
Get More Done
in Less Time

With great precision, I plan everything in advance:
who's dropping off, who's picking up. We have charts,
maps, and lists on the fridge, all over the house.
I sometimes feel like I'm in the CIA.

— KATE WINSLET,
on the question of balancing work and raising two kids

Good time management can change your life. If you've heard it once, you've heard it a million times—but there's good reason. One of the biggest energy drainers that moms fail to address is poor time management. And this can have a serious impact on your energy. Planning your meals, grocery shopping, basic errands, personal time, and house cleaning—just generally keeping everything afloat—takes a lot of effort. Is there an ideal way to map out a week? We think so, and it doesn't have to resemble your mother's cookie-cutter plans or any other mother's for that matter. It just has to match your habits, lifestyle, and personal needs.

Years ago, Stephen R. Covey was made famous for his quadrant theory on what makes a highly effective individual, which became a cornerstone in his *First Things First* and *The 7 Habits of Highly Effective People* bestsellers. He revolutionized the business world, changing how executives, managers, and even everyday people allocate their time and accomplish goals. Covey created his masterpiece long before we had the Internet at our fingertips, chronic e-mails blasting through to us and competing for brain space, and more digital junk than we know what to do with. His Time Management Matrix is undoubtedly more relevant today than ever.

Well, we've taken Covey's matrix and modified it so it's attuned to a mother's needs and demands. We're calling it the Energy Matrix. Where you see yourself in this matrix says a lot about your energy woes—and how to fix them.

> **Profile Alert!** Although the information in this chapter will benefit all the profile types, people who saw themselves as fitting Profile 2 (The Mom Zombie), Profile 3 (The Overworked and Overscheduled), and Profile 5 (The Dead Battery) should pay particular attention here.

THE ENERGY MATRIX

Which Quadrant defines the kind of life you're living? Ask yourself where your priorities are. When something comes across your desk as "urgent," how do you respond? What brings you stress and feelings of being overwhelmed? Are you a master at excuses, a proactive leader in your life, or just dead in the water? Let's find out.

Which of the following sets of descriptions best relates to you?

Quadrant I: Urgent and Important

If you're living in Quadrant I, everything seems urgent and important. Your life is about crisis, pressing problems, and deadline-driven projects.

How many of the following boxes can you check?

☐ I respond immediately to everyone and everything, and am constantly putting out fires.

☐ I live with extreme energy highs and lows, and feel anxious all the time—I'm constantly in crisis mode.

☐ I don't make To Do lists and have never been good with priorities.

Examples of life in Quad I: Ringing phone, crying child, last-minute bill paying, backloading (eating the majority of your calories in the back half of the day), trying every fad diet but getting no results, and abusing short-term energy fillers such as caffeine and sugar.

Symptoms of too much living in Quad I: Overwhelming stress, extreme energy highs and lows, weight gain, anxiety, sleeplessness, fatigue, mood swings, arguments with others, carb cravings, high blood pressure, high anxiety, heart palpitations, digestive problems, headaches, no major accomplishments, nonexistent sex life, no time to do anything you love, grabbing the bottle of wine before happy hour ("Hey, it's happy hour somewhere"), canceling your personal appointments that make you feel like a woman, unhappiness, dissatisfaction.

Bottom line: You're *reactive* rather than *proactive*.

Quadrant II: Not Urgent but Important

A mom in Quadrant II works hard at self-development and health maintenance. She also works at building her relationships and planning smartly for the future. This is the sweet-spot Quadrant where life feels relatively balanced and rarely are there issues about lack of energy.

How many of the following boxes can you check?

☐ I'm a pretty good planner and map out my days—even my future years—carefully. I'm also good about planning my meals and "me" time, so that I get what I need to get done, eat well, and find peace with myself.

☐ I rarely feel deprived because I take responsibility for my choices and practice discipline.

☐ I share deep connections with others, feel energetic most of the time, and enjoy the thrill of learning something new.

Examples of life in Quad II: Exercise, recreation, learning about nutrition and what feeds you, fulfillment, education/developing new skills, planning meals, scheduling events and personal time-outs, date night, weekly dinner with friends, vacations, hobbies, setting goals for future, relaxation techniques, playing with the kids, crafting, meditation, magazine time, physical contact with others (massage, facial, acupuncture, reflexology), making choices so you don't feel deprived (e.g., you might choose to have dessert at one point, or wine, etc. but you're at energy harmony so your choices are coming from what you know is best, whether it's indulging or choosing not to).

The blissful signs of living in Quad II: Balance, discipline, hope for the future, deep connections with others, an ideal weight, feeling energetic and well rested, in control of one's life, happiness, feeling that life is good.

Bottom line: You're *proactive* and life is good.

Quadrant III: Urgent but Not Important

You know what it's like to live in Quadrant III if you let everything steal your attention and walk over you even if it's not necessarily important. Interruptions and unscheduled phone calls are the norm. You let trivial mail and pointless meetings distract you. You constantly address things that can wait, and feel depleted on a regular basis for doing so.

How many of the following boxes can you check?

☐ I stay up late catching up on important tasks that I didn't accomplish during the day because of all the "busy work."

☐ I have an endless texting plan and use up my minutes every month.

☐ I hate myself for failing at another diet and blame my demanding kids and boss for not letting me succeed.

Examples of life in Quad III: Responding to e-mails that can wait, accepting/making phone calls that can wait, going to every single PTA or community meeting, saying yes to things you really don't care about or can delegate to someone else, saying yes because you feel guilty, comparing yourself to others, not making priorities, chronic dieting, excuses galore.

Symptoms of too much living in Quad III: Feeling victimized, out of control, unmotivated, and deprived. You sense that goals and plans are worthless because you never get the results you want.

Bottom line: You're *reactive* but rather than a victim of immediate pressing circumstances, you're just not being strategic enough for your needs. You're not thinking long term, and you lack focus. Everything feels too hard, too difficult. There are *a lot of excuses* in this category.

Quadrant IV: Not Urgent and Not Important

Do you fall into the trap of doing busywork? The hallmarks of Quad IV include a lot of time wasters that don't enhance your life (or your energy). Maybe it's the pull of the television or Internet, or the addiction to shopping for no apparent reason (and without a list). Or maybe it's an obsession with your smartphone, as you check e-mail and messages as if you're in the midst of a serious crisis, and you cannot go a day without texting. Routines and schedules are not your thing, and you have no idea where to begin to prioritize your life because it's become such a shapeless blob of craziness.

How many of the following boxes can you check?

☐ I take care of things when I feel like it, even if that means someone else suffers, a bill is late getting paid, or I have to lose a night of sleep and eat crap because I haven't gone to the grocery store.

☐ Stuff tends to pile up quickly at home, but I'm not motivated to clear it out.

☐ I feel emotionally bankrupt, have wondered if I'm depressed, and have no idea what to expect of myself in the future.

Examples of life in Quad IV: Endless/mindless TV watching (and channel surfing) or Internet surfing, late-night e-mailing and Web browsing/blog reading, reading junk mail/e-mail, goalless shopping, engaging in conversation with toxic people, doing the dishes/cleaning house after your preferred bedtime.

Symptoms of too much living in Quad IV: Lacking a routine, unconscious eating and food obsessions, disconnectedness with yourself and others. You let yourself go and feel emotionally empty. You lack a sense of responsibility and are unable to meet bigger, long-term goals for you and your family.

Bottom line: You're *inactive*. Inert. Indifferent. You watch the exercise video or *The Biggest Loser* TV show but you're not connected to yourself enough to take action. You're living outside your own body. Your kids (and spouse) want to fire you!

The Mom Energy Matrix

Quad I: Urgent and Important

- Living in crisis mode
- Pressing problems
- Deadline-driven projects

You respond to everything in the moment and live on stimulants such as caffeine and sugar. You seek quick fixes but never get the results you want in any area of your life. To say you run low on energy all the time is an understatement.

You're *reactive* rather than *proactive*.

Quad II: Not Urgent but Important

- Focusing on self-development and health maintenance
- Relationship building
- Planning the future

You're in control of your life and have energy harmony. Even in the face of unexpected challenges and energy suckers, you find a way to maintain balance because you're well prepared.

You're *proactive* and life is good.

Quad III: Urgent but Not Important

- Interruptions, unscheduled phone calls
- Distracting mail and meetings
- Things that can wait

You struggle with goals and agendas. Everything seems high-priority and you let it take over your life. When something fails, you find an excuse to cover for it. Your life lacks structure. Keeping all the balls in the air—especially ones you shouldn't be carrying—are constantly draining your energy. Finding new excuses is also depleting.

You're *reactive* and full of excuses. You lack focus and structure.

Quad IV: Not Urgent and Not Important

- Busywork
- Time wasters
- Addictions and obsessions

You are the quintessential mom who has let herself go. Nothing takes priority, not even you when you need it most. You are running on empty—and don't have a clue where to begin. You can't acknowledge your nonexistent energy because you're out of touch and can't read the signals your body is telling you.

You're *inactive*. Inert. Indifferent. If you knew how bad it was, you'd fire yourself.

In which category did you find yourself? Are you playing the victim (Quad I), living in reactive mode (Quad III), acting as if you're dead (Quad IV), or really being proactive (Quad II)? If you've got energy issues, then we doubt you're living a proactive life today. Our guess is that most of you are hanging out in Quad I, III, or IV and wishing you were in Quad II. It's perfectly normal to find yourself hovering somewhere between Quadrants and see yourself with a mix of descriptors from all categories. Hybrids of these Quads are possible, and if there's one common denominator for those living mostly in Quad I, III, or IV, it's a lack of prioritizing and creating realistic To Do lists attuned to your true vision and needs.

Take a deep breath. We don't expect any mom to feel as if she has to always thrive in Quad II. That's unrealistic. All of us inhabit each of these Quads in the real world. Life happens. Kids get sick, and you get tired. The difference between what's "urgent" or "important" can be fuzzy or can suddenly change. The goal is to learn to recognize where you are within these Quadrants, and with that awareness, optimize your situation so you don't have to let the circumstances or consequences affect you as much. In other words, don't let yourself remain a victim or be inactive for too long. If you're stuck in Quad I, III, or IV for whatever reason, make it a goal to shift out quicker than the last time you inhabited that place. By the same token, we know it's not fair to tell a new mom, a menopausal woman, or a mom with three teens that she has to plan everything or focus on relationship building. But we want to show you how to avoid being totally unprepared and blindsided by the serious repercussions of not taking control of your time. There will be moments when you need to put a relationship in a holding pattern, and that's okay. At the end of the day, we're shooting for your health and your energy—no one else's!

No matter who you are—whether you're a working or stay-at-home mom—there's never enough time to finish all the To Dos.

Everyone has a list of things to do that exceeds the physical limitations of time and boundless energy. The concept of free time just doesn't exist for anyone these days. But here's another way to look at it. You say you don't have time, but considering that lacking energy prevents us from capitalizing on our time, imagine all the time you'll magically create by just getting this one area in your life under control.

Time is no longer something I have anymore.
I realized to live the lifestyle and have the profession I have,
I needed to prioritize how I get my energy and use it wisely. . . .
I have a huge problem doing two things at once and getting
either one done fully. Now that I am a mom, I find it almost
a necessity to be able to do two things at the same time
to get anything done. How do I do that?

— JESSICA MENDOZA,
professional softball player, Women's Sports Foundation
president, and ESPN commentator

The Secrets to Sanity

Shifting into Quadrant II won't happen overnight. It will take patience, consistency, and a shift in thinking as much as a shift in lifestyle. We don't know any mom who isn't time-crunched and on the verge of burnout, but it doesn't have to be that way.

The solution? Develop a system for organizing your life according to what needs to get done now, what can wait until later, and what can wait until much later. Use this system for everything that demands your attention during the day, whether it's a phone call, an unhappy child, or a piece of mail. Prioritize your tasks by creating To Dos marked "now," "later," and "can wait." Set standards for dealing with important monthly stuff, such as bills, by designating every other Sunday to address the unpaid bills or mail that requires your attention within a certain time period.

If you're the reactive type who's easily distracted, then you may want to create boundaries for yourself by checking e-mail, watching television, and turning on your cell-phone ringer during only certain hours of the day. For some people, mornings before ten o'clock can be an incredibly efficient pocket of time for taking care of important tasks. This may be when you choose to catch up with your sister, or complete urgent or routine tasks such as tidying up your living quarters or balancing your checkbook.

The following strategies can help you make the shift into living in Quad II. Incorporate as many as you can into your life. Take them one at a time if you need to, adding more strategies each week or month as necessary.

Track your life: There are lots of habits that people get into without realizing it. Take a few days—or even a week—at a time to record everything you do. Keep track of what time you go to bed and when you wake up. Also include how many times you wake up in the night. Do you get up? Why do you get up? How long do you stay awake? Do you have lots of electronic lights on in the room? Do noises keep you awake? What clothes do you wear to bed? Do you watch TV before falling asleep? The answers to these questions may ultimately relate to your energy shortages.

Keep a chart for your exercise workouts and the duration of each one. See how consistent you are with keeping a routine, as this plays a huge role in your energy. This is a good exercise for moms in any Quad. We all have lows in energy during the day, and it's important to know when that low arrives and what you habitually do about it. Tracking your life to know where your time goes— down to every last minute—will help you to implement other strategies for organizing your life and planning accordingly.

Take inventory of your Band-Aids: This is also a good exercise for any mom. Examine your diet and medicine cabinet for the culprits: fast food, energy bars, mochaccinos, pain and headache medication, acid reflux/digestive medication, prepackaged foods, soda, and sleeping pills. Try to manage these better. You may need some of these once in a while, but not every day. Highly reactive and inactive people tend to rely on medications and exterior sources of "energy" to keep going.

Distinguish between urgent and important: Anyone who found herself in Quad I or III should do this on everything, from your son's principal calling to your husband's pleas for attention. "Urgent" refers to things that truly have an immediate impact on you and your family's health and life, such as a sick child. However, consider that the urgent shouldn't always take precedence over the important. It's easy to let emergencies or the latest crisis run your day, and if you don't develop the skill of knowing when the important trumps the urgent, you won't ever be in control—because you'll be chasing after the urgent and ignoring what's important. Identify those tasks that truly need your attention first, and don't allow yourself to be distracted. Just because someone puts one of those high-priority flags on their e-mail doesn't automatically make it so. Prioritize. Prioritize. Prioritize and manage your day accordingly.

I try to be aware and stay on top of all my challenges one day and sometimes one hour at a time. I take it one thing at a time, first things first, and then go from there.

— CHAKA KHAN,

ten-time Grammy Award–winning singer, songwriter,
philanthropist, mother, and grandmother

Structure your day and take control of every minute: Don't let incoming work control you. It bears repeating: set boundaries—specific time periods during which certain tasks get completed while other, less important tasks wait. If you're prone to distractions such as e-mail, phone, or the television, put a system in place for blocking out these intrusions and addressing them only during certain times of the day. This may mean checking e-mail only once every four hours, or allowing the television to be on during specified time periods. While moms in all Quads would do well to follow this advice, inhabitants of Quad IV should pay particular attention. Structure will help you to manage your busywork and place importance on things that are indeed important. Structure will also give you the motivation and inspiration to take charge in ways that will pull you out of a miserably inactive, inert, and indifferent life. You'll begin to feel happier and more in control, too.

Get control of your paperwork: Create a mail center, where all mail goes and gets dealt with. In this same place, set up a message center containing a calendar marked with important dates. Hang a whiteboard to jot down important lists, To Dos, or that thought you don't want to lose. Try a corkboard, too, to pin those circulars, notices, or invitations that you don't want to forget.

Assign a specific day to prioritize and plan: This gets you into the habit of scheduling food and workouts around non-negotiable commitments; maybe you can get other family members involved and divvy up responsibilities. Set a time and day for laundry, food shopping, meal planning, house cleanup, and so on. Typically a Sunday is the ultimate day to prioritize. Make sure that you spend some time looking ahead at what's coming so you can prep yourself. Note the pitfalls: the two-hour parent-teacher night that tends to last three hours; the regular Thursday staff meeting; the 85 unanswered e-mails that could consume the entire morning. Every day has its molehills, but if you're prepared and limit the time you give them, they won't turn into mountains. Know your appointments and commitments, but look at them in terms of where you're going to schedule workouts, "me" time, and obligations you want to keep for yourself. For example, Tuesdays and Fridays could be your 5:30 A.M. workouts while Wednesdays are the day you'll exercise after the kids go to bed. When you have a realistic plan in your head and on your calendar, chances are you'll follow it closely. You'll feel in control and manage to fit everything in *and* have room for the unexpected. You may, for instance, hit a week where you realize that there are three nights that you cannot make dinner for your family. Knowing this in advance allows you to plan accordingly; maybe that first night will be Crock-Pot dinner, with leftovers the next night.

At first I thought I could not give as much energy as was demanded. It was overwhelming . . . but then I adapted . . . I had to adjust and learn to prioritize my time . . . start my day with silence to find my balance and end it with a little R & R to regain my sanity. One must stay focused and delegate time to different projects as needed. When I start my day in silence, this gives me the focus I need to organize the rest of my day efficiently.

— MARIEL HEMINGWAY,

mother, author, yogi, and spokesperson for green living

Go online: Pay your bills and monitor your financial accounts online wherever you can. For help with all things organization, try Google Calendar. Experiment with online grocery shopping. Some major chains now offer free delivery, and once you have a trusty list of staples, you can double-click your way to a full, healthy kitchen. Imagine the time saved! You can spend that extra time on just *you*.

Practice IKEA-style cooking (i.e., some assembly required): While we'll discuss more of the specifics of food choice in the upcoming chapters, one big part of time management focuses on cooking and shopping, so we have to mention this strategy here. Keep healthy ingredients on hand that can be assembled into a variety of delicious dishes. Aside from your usual shopping routine, schedule a trip to the grocery store once every three or four months when you can spend some time investigating labels or to check out a new market—farmers' or regular. This trial-and-error time will help you comfortably expand and maximize your future time.

Don't let your kids be enablers: We've hinted at it before and we'll stress this again, because it's one of the most pervasive problems facing moms today. Kids afford moms the perfect excuse to buy all kinds of junk and, let's face it, avoid exercise. We watch so many moms go through the motions of a day like this: being "good" in the morning by limiting calories with coffee and/or a diet-conscious smoothie or bar for breakfast, then a salad with chicken for lunch, which then progresses to nibbling on the kids' after-school snacks and cookies, skipping a workout to tidy up the house and perform chores, downing mac and cheese, pasta, or fast food with the kids for dinner . . . and then letting loose in the kitchen late at night once the kids have gone to bed. Sound familiar?

Don't feed the cycle: When TV, bills, and Internet call late at night, a mom can easily wind up feeling revved up with enough anxiety and a rush of sugar from that last bowl of ice cream to avert bedtime. So what does she do? Pop a sleep aid and then feel guilty about staying up too late, which then affects her energy the following day. The vicious cycle continues. A mom in reactive mode (Quad I or III) can find herself in this cycle at any given time. Be aware of it. See what you can do to seize control of it.

Make big goals smaller: Listen up, moms in Quad IV, who feel so overwhelmed by everything that you're seemingly paralyzed and inactive! If you can't seem to ever get anything done, maybe your goals are just too big or unrealistic. Persistently pursuing a big dream is great when you're getting somewhere. But if you're not, it's the energy-draining pits. Repeatedly hitting dead ends can also make your levels of CRP— C-reactive protein, a marker of inflammation—rise. Since inflammation has been linked to depressive symptoms, stewing over going nowhere may add to your blues. Instead, let go of what's not working and replace it with smaller, newer, more reachable goals.

Take a 10-minute mind-trip: Remember the last time you were on vacation and it embodied every definition of that word? You can go there any time you like—and reap the relaxing rewards—using your imagination. All it takes is a quiet spot, an easy chair or place to lie down, and 10 to 15 uninterrupted minutes. Eyes closed, bring to your mind an image of the place where you felt peaceful and happy. Now scan the scene from top to bottom, left to right and "see" little details—the way the sun reflected off the water or the appearance of a decadent dinner. What sounds did you hear? How did the air smell? Relive as many things as you can. Feel the pure pleasure of being in that space and time. You'll soon feel as relaxed as if you'd actually been there. You can then open your eyes and be prepared to maximize your time and energy better. Moms who live in Quad II already know how to enjoy their mental time-outs, and anyone seeking to join them can master this technique as well.

I really think that television is a total energy suck. Sometimes it's great to just veg out and give in to that, but I think it should be something that we look forward to once in a while—rather than every day. Even if you just have it on in the background, the sound and visual movement on TV interrupts the kind of focus you need to foster in order to get things done as a mom. We have enough little energy suckers running around, let's limit the ones we can turn off!

— RACHEL LINCOLN SARNOFF,

executive director and CEO of Healthy Child Healthy World, founder of www.EcoStiletto.com, and mom of three, on secrets to energy success

---

Listen to your body: It sounds cliché, but it's true. Listening to your body can do wonders, and you know what kind of listening we're talking about. It's the kind that dictates a mother's instincts. It's also the kind that allows you to be really honest with yourself and your needs, avoiding excuses, external messages or influences that can block your ability to hear yourself. When you're contemplating exercise, for instance, you can say, "C'mon, are you just feeling lazy and sorry for yourself? Overwhelmed? That's when you need to pull yourself up by your bootstraps and go! You'll get so much from it." We know how to listen to our bodies. We are women. We've been listening since our training bras. We're far better at this than men. Don't fool yourself or use excuses.

Becoming a master of time management takes more than practice. It also takes a commitment every single day to navigating competing demands and constantly asking yourself where you should be putting your energy first, second, third, and so on. Most of us let our time-management skills fall by the wayside once in a while, even those of us who think we're living in Quad II. It's inevitable. We intuitively know what's really urgent and what's not but we feel compelled to respond to everything. And there's no end to the amount of information we increasingly find ourselves bombarded with through e-mail, snail mail, texts, IM, the television, and so on.

Just having a good sense of where your weaknesses are and keeping practical strategies on hand will help you to get through your days with efficiency, and hopefully some energy left over. We hope the lessons in this chapter will prepare you for the advice coming up in the next two chapters on making "energy exchanges" in your dietary choices. We don't know any mother who doesn't waste precious time trying to keep up with all the myriad choices we have now in the marketplace. Between the promotional machines and the sheer number of options in the grocery stores, it can get downright confusing and exhausting. So, in addition to reorganizing your time and priorities, let's now turn to how you can rethink your grocery shopping and, in turn, reorganize your kitchen, pantries, and entire eating patterns.

MOM UP! JUMP-START YOUR TRANSFORMATION

Regardless of which Quadrant you're in, see if you can up your level of productivity and overall energy just doing the following: go on a media purge for one week. This means being brutal with the time you spend on the Internet, e-mail, and television. Set very clear boundaries, such as not checking e-mail or doing anything digitally related until after 10 A.M. On the other end of the day, disconnect yourself from electronics at 6 P.M. to spend quality time with the family. Try to avoid reading too many headlines as well. Author Timothy Ferriss writes about going on such a purge in his best-selling book *The 4-Hour Workweek* (if only motherhood held such a promise!), and he proves how enormously transformative it can be to a person's overall ability to get things done (with energy to spare). So see if you can last for one full week on a media purge and take note of how you feel (better) and what you're able to accomplish (more). This is like giving your body a time-management "reboot"—you'll emerge out of the purge with a new perspective on what's really important and be able to better prioritize and manage your life. You'll lose the fat (life in Quads I, III, and IV) and gain the fitness (life in Quad II).

CHAPTER 4

The Energy Exchange Part 1: Ditch Energy Drainers in Your Diet

Motherhood has a very humanizing effect.
Everything gets reduced to essentials.

— M E R Y L   S T R E E P

We live in an age where dietary advice comes at us from every portal of our daily lives. Some of these new advancements fall under the high-tech category, such as keeping a food journal on our phones or scanning a bar code for additional info or ratings on food products. Other high-tech advancements fall into the arena of food technology. Food product developers can now make seemingly healthier versions of our favorite foods by adding artificial scents and tastes that remind us of the original thing. They can also use chemicals such as artificial preservatives and additives, as well as pesticides and genetic engineering of plant and possibly animal DNA.

We've gone from living in a primal forest where our food was picked directly from the ground or plucked from trees to living in a technologically advanced Jetsons-style society where even our "natural" foods are engineered. To think we can engineer animals now, such as salmon, to "create" fish that are twice the size in half the time is amazing on the one hand, but on the other raises questions. Is this a good thing? What does eating a genetically modified fish do to our bodies?

If we think that speeding up the growth process could have any positive merits, then let's think about what else involves sped-up cells: cancer and premature aging, anyone? And what does it mean for developmental stages among consumers of genetically modified foods that may (or may not) adversely affect our biology? When we take shortcuts, there are usually trade-offs to consider. And when it comes to genetically modified foods, we just don't know yet what repercussions could be brewing. Eating foods that look normal on the outside could be telling another story on the inside. Added hormones in the food chain have already been blamed for some of the trends in adolescents whereby girls reach puberty much sooner than girls in previous generations.

So while all this food technology makes our food prettier and bigger, it also departs from nature. These foods don't necessarily speak our bodies' native language, which means they can throw our energy equations off balance. When it comes to foods, consider the watchful phrase "just because they can doesn't mean we should."

As much as the world around us has vastly changed, our bodies still speak the same basic language they have always and forever known. But now the ingredients listed on the packaging of foods often sound more like an advanced chemistry lesson than a simple snack. And just as these words sound foreign to us, our bodies aren't naturally programmed to understand "monosodium glutamate," either. When we lived in the state of nature, there was a perfect fit between our physiology and our food supply. What we ate was perfectly suited to our physical needs—and as a result we "hummed." Chronic low energy and a sedentary baseline would have been completely unknown to our primitive ancestors. Obviously, we are not recommending that we all don loincloths and try to recapture the primeval lifestyle, but we could learn a lot from our cavewoman ancestors. Think about it: without lights they went to bed and rose with the sun. Energy wasn't an option; it was a means of survival.

PREPARE TO END BODY CHAOS: GO BACK TO HIGH SCHOOL

You remember the days when life was relatively easy. You got up, went to school, probably did something fun afterward, and then sat down to do homework before going to bed to rest up for another day. Your choices in snacks were probably healthier than they are today, too, by virtue of the fact we didn't have so many processed options back then. Thoughts about the "real world" and having children were farther away than your dreams. The kind of math you were trying to understand was something along the lines of $a + b = c$.

You may have forgotten algebra now that you are, in fact, in the real world, but the beauty and simplicity with which algebra allows us to make certain calculations can be applied to our biology. Metaphorically speaking, that is. When you treat your body in simple, straightforward terms, it will respond by maximizing functionality and energy production. When you feed it "fake" ingredients, suddenly $a + b$ no longer equals c. Instead, we get a $1 + b + 2 = c1 + 2$. Body chaos ensues. The energy equation breaks down. This is what lays the foundation for chronic disease and blocks energy.

Nutritional medicine is a rapidly growing area of research that will continue to gain momentum as we learn more and more about the connections between nutrition and health—not just for general health, but for all kinds of health concerns. In fact, the link between nutrition and diseases such as obesity, diabetes, cancer, and cardiovascular disease are well documented. Gaining the upper hand on oxidative stress, inflammation, and, to a lesser extent, genetics, is key because they are the chief agers in our bodies that spur chronic conditions that wear us down. And if diet can help this in any way, then we should be paying attention.

Anything that goes against the natural design of our body's most basic and elemental needs will invariably sabotage efforts to maximize energy. For example, that diet soda or latte may work as a (very) short-term fix, but it will only exacerbate the problems that are underlying your energy shortage. Similarly, if you're conscientiously following a diet program that isn't operating in sync with your body's true needs, then no matter how "good" you're being or how saintly your intent, you are not going to see the results you are working so hard to obtain.

We realize that you may have heard (and tried) to "avoid processed foods" in the past to drop a few pounds or get healthier. But your efforts eventually failed. We agree, it can be daunting and ultimately unsatisfying, as well as unrealistic. We live in the 21st century, and there's something to be said for having access to quick and great-tasting food. We're not asking you to nix everything that hails from a factory or comes in a package. We're just asking you to manage the energy drainers in your life by (1) recognizing where they are, and (2) being more mindful of how much you choose to pick from the energy-giving plate versus the energy-sapping one. And therein lies the challenge: knowing the difference between what you think you're eating and what you really are. Today's marketing dynamics are just as much to blame in perpetuating body chaos as we are to blame for favoring processed foods over wholesome, natural ones.

Modifying the way you eat and buy goods may take some time to get used to. We won't sugarcoat the reality: if you've been eating processed, packaged foods regularly for years, shifting how you eat won't happen overnight. And that's okay. Make it a goal to just upgrade at a pace that's doable and with choices that give you the biggest nutritional bang for your food buck. If you can't imagine changing your breakfast or lunch staples, then what about adding organic vegetables to them? What about swapping out a less-healthy fat for a healthier one in your dressing? What about splitting your meal in half and having the second part three hours later for better energy balance? What if these evolutions, not revolutions, resulted in more energy, looser-fitting clothes, and an internally healthier you? We can confidently say they can and will. We've found the weight-loss factor in particular to be enormously motivating for women. In fact, both of us have witnessed women who simply stopped using coffee creamers and artificially flavored beverages (sold under the guise of "light" or "diet" items) and achieved significant results in just a week's time. And they far outpace those who go back to consuming artificial ingredients in their weight-loss efforts. Keep it simple, and the body gets it and has an easier time getting rid of excess fat, not to mention toxins that go with it.

If the thought of depriving yourself of the foods you currently enjoy doesn't sit well with you, then simply pick up more fresh fruits and vegetables at the market and don't change anything else. Make additions rather than deletions to your lifestyle at the start. You can and will wean yourself from the stuff the real energy is not made of once you begin to incorporate nutrient-dense, energy-supporting alternatives into your life. Over time, when you aren't operating from a self-deprivation strategy, you will notice that your taste buds have changed and you'll find yourself obsessing less over the displays at the bakery and more over what you can do with the colorful array of goods in the produce section of a market. Or as one mom-energy model shared with me: "We get a delivery now once a week of organic vegetables so we've had to get creative about how to use them. I love the recipes they send, but I have also started swapping with some friends on Facebook who get the same vegetable box." As with anything, as you become comfortable with it, your priorities change and you begin to instinctively make different choices. (Does this remind you of other big changes you've already gone through in your life as a mom?) You'll start to order food differently in a restaurant and be more conscious about reading labels and asking questions about how your meals are prepared.

In recent years, we learned to "skip the center and shop the perimeter" of the food market, but as we learned and changed our shopping behaviors, so did the stores and the companies. Today, the perimeter often has as much poor-quality food on display as the healthy stuff. If we can't trust the package and we can't shop the perimeter, does this mean there are no shortcuts to healthy shopping and hence healthy eating? Does shopping have to be a new skill that we must study to achieve successfully? Well, yes and no. Before you close the book and shudder at the thought of more to do, exhale and read on to our list of shortcuts—but also note that changing habits and learning new things does require a commitment. But just like you don't run a mile the first day you decide to exercise, you can start by walking—and walking through the grocery store means taking a list based on the ideas and examples in this book and trying to replace the items that you would have bought before with healthier versions to see how it goes. It may feel boring or limiting, but it will be safe. It will save you time. It will get you results. And then as you succeed, you can start to increase your speed, add hills, run for longer—or the equivalent in the grocery store by trying to modify old favorites.

One prominent food manufacturer once promoted its brand by challenging children to recite the ingredients in a popular product. The kids who read the label could clearly state—and understand—the words, such as *eggs* and *milk*. The kids who read the competition stumbled over long, convoluted ingredients that sounded like a chemistry set. The lesson: if you can easily pronounce the words on a list of ingredients, nine times out of ten you're eating something close to nature. That's a pretty good barometer to use.

When you walk into the fresh produce department of a grocery store, you're not likely to find "high in vitamin C" on an orange, or "a great source of healthy fats" on an avocado. Instead, these claims are trumpeted from boxed, processed, and packaged goods.

Whenever a processed product boasts such a claim, you should question why. Food manufacturers want to control what matters to you. Every single food and food product in the store has a marketing team working hard to promote the brand. The net effect: when you walk down a grocery aisle, it's like hundreds of voices talking to you at one time (and you thought a household with two to five voices could get crazy). It's overstimulation, and we need to take our brains back! Let's look at some considerations:

- Even if a manufacturer has added something to a food to achieve a higher nutritional level than what exists in nature, it begs the question: is the form of what's added absorbable? Can we absorb that much? Should we? What's the rationale?

- Just because manufacturers can and do add nutrients to a food product, does that action have other consequences, such as competing with what's naturally in the food? For example, increasingly higher calcium in the absence of magnesium can create an imbalance of these two minerals that ultimately detracts from your body's energy-making machine.

- If we give too much attention to one vitamin, can it create a "conditional deficiency" of another? (Ask your kids: if you give more attention to one, how does the other feel?) B vitamins work best together, so if we over support one B vitamin, we can create a condition whereby the lack of others at the same level creates unhealthy byproducts and dysenergy—dysfunctional energy—issues in the body. Whom do we trust to meet our nutrient needs: Mother Manufacturer or Mother Nature?

- What about getting 100 percent (or more) of your daily needs in one food—is that a smart goal? At first it seems great because it means we don't have to think about getting any more throughout the day, but we should think about consuming nutrients all day long, especially from whole-food sources. A glass of OJ at breakfast with 100 percent of your daily vitamin C needs doesn't mean you should shun a real orange or other vitamin C–packed whole fruit later on as part of a snack.

- And what about ingredients added to foods that naturally wouldn't contain them? For example, our yogurt may not supply us with a lot of fiber, but it gives us high-quality protein plus pre- and probiotics—the ingredients to support lean body mass, a healthy balance of hormones, digestive wellness, and heightened immunity. We can increase fiber by adding fresh fruit or ground flaxseed on top. Yogurts that add synthetic or processed fibers may be less than ideal, but moreover, they are unnecessary when you rely on nature's fiber sources.

Don't judge a book by its cover: The front of all packaged goods simply reflects what you told the food manufacturers you want. Yes, we all want a high-fiber, low-sugar, low-fat, delicious combination of ingredients that will cure cancer, provide energy, and help us fit into our skinny clothes. But always be sure to check the nutrition facts and ingredients. Just because the front of the package says so, doesn't mean the contents can or will deliver.

Marketing terms are regulated but to date, unfortunately, not very well enforced, and again, these terms aren't typically a complete nutrition thought. For example, "Naturally fat free" could distract us from the fact the product is loaded with sugar. Deceptive claims abound: low-fat, high-fiber, light, no sugar added. Some brands have become more healthful. But many manufacturers are promoting a product's healthful ingredients while playing down its less nutritional qualities. Last year, the FDA sent warning letters to 17 food manufacturers, many of which were household names, insisting they change the wording on their labels. Even First Lady Michelle Obama and the White House Task Force on Childhood Obesity have recommended that labeling on food packages be more clearly defined, yet they believe it should come from the companies regulating themselves. Companies respond to consumer demand, so in order for them to self-regulate we need to demand that change by buying differently. In 2010, the Center for Science in the Public Interest, a nonprofit health-advocacy organization, published an alarming report called "Food Labeling Chaos" about just that—the confusion over what labels claim. The changes currently being lobbied about in Washington, D.C., could take years to go into effect. Until then, be wary of the words and phrases you're reading in the grocery aisles. Here's our cheat sheet to the marketing mayhem.

Natural or organic: One is legally regulated, the other is a marketing concept with no definition. A company can use the term *natural* to mean just about anything. Consumers often assume it implies organic, but that's not the case. The U.S. Department of Agriculture has strict guidelines for a company to meet before it can label a food organic, but the organic versus nonorganic conversation can sometimes get confusing. (We'll discuss more on the term *organic* later.)

Made with whole wheat: If it does not say 100 percent whole wheat or 100 percent whole grain, then be wary. The food may contain only a trivial amount of whole grain. Example: one popular brand of English muffins lists "unbleached enriched wheat flour" as its primary ingredient. That is just a fancy phrase for ordinary white flour.

Healthy: To use the word *healthy,* companies must meet certain FDA regulations per serving size. Some companies have been accused of increasing the number of serving sizes per product, rather than change the ingredients. If a person eats the entire jar or drinks the whole bottle, it would not meet the regulations. Manipulating the serving size is, by some experts, the most dangerous problem in food-labeling confusion. We've all eaten an entire can of soup thinking it's all one serving. But if you look closely, the nutrition label on the back might say otherwise—and it may even list a strange 2.5 servings for two and a half people. So at the end of the can, you've downed more than twice the number of calories and probably maxed out your sodium needs for the entire day—not a good thing for balance and energy. Remember, a food shouldn't have to tell you what it is—as in "healthy" or "food"—so if it does, then it likely isn't telling you the whole story, but rather telling you *their* story. It should be illegal for companies to use words such as *healthy, lean,* or *light* unless those foods adhere to a clear set of nutrition principles. In England, for example, food manufacturers aren't allowed to use the term *superfood* without meeting certain science-based criteria. Clearly, such terms have a lot of marketing power.

Supports or a source of: These are loose terms that insinuate the food helps protect against a popular health concern. The latest trend is a lack of vitamin D, because of concerns that a deficiency in vitamin D may play a role in a host of health conditions, from obesity to dementia and even autism. If a food says it is an "excellent source of vitamin D," it may only mean that it will provide a percentage of the current RDA, which is 600 IU (International Units). However, most experts agree the current RDA is extremely low for general health, as well as completely insufficient to replenish those who are clinically low in vitamin D. Moreover, you could be getting it in a form that isn't well absorbed. D is a fat-soluble vitamin, so it helps to have some healthy fat nearby to ensure optimal absorption.

High in fiber: Dietary fiber is critical to a healthy diet and the proper functioning of our bodies. It helps our bodies absorb carbohydrates efficiently; it help us feel full; it aids digestion both by adding bulk to stool and by scraping the lining of the digestive tract (our built-in cleaning system); it aids heart health; and as a prebiotic, it promotes a hospitable environment for probiotics, the healthy bacteria that help our digestion and support our immune system. Although fiber is not technically a nutrient, its role in managing the nutrients in your body—and its energy equations—is so essential to your health and metabolism that we might as well call it a nutrient.

Fiber is naturally found in the skins of fruits and vegetables, legumes, sprouts, and grains (especially whole grains). Most people don't get enough fiber, which is in the orbit of at least 25 grams per day for women. Our consumption of highly processed foods and beverages (other than pure water) has decreased the average amount of fiber in our collective diet; as a result, numerous synthetic fibers are sold as supplements and added into food products. Is the fiber found in a processed box of sugary cereal the same as what drops from an apple tree? Not nearly.

Many foods contain "isolated fibers" to boost the fiber content. But it is unlikely these isolated fibers, usually inulin, polydextrose, and maltodextrin, provide the same health benefits as "intact fibers," such as those found in whole beans or oats. Fiber One Oats & Chocolate bars, for instance, provide 35 percent of daily fiber, but the fiber comes mainly from chicory root extract, which contains inulin, and which incidentally can cause bloating and gas in many when they consume significant quantities at one time.

While these additives may add bulk and provide some of fiber's benefits, they don't necessarily include the phytonutrients, vitamins, and minerals found in nature's fiber sources. Add whole foods into your diet first, and then carefully incorporate fiber-added products only as needed. Try to include some fiber at every meal. If you have food allergies or intolerances, it's important for you to include other natural sources of fiber (rice bran, chia bran, and flaxseeds are excellent sources) to make up for the fib r in the foods you avoid. And watch out for fiber added to foods that are high in sugar. Froot Loops, for example, says it "now provides fiber." But the 12 grams of sugar in each 1 cup serving of the cereal could have far more negative effects than any benefit from the slim amount of added fiber.

Zero trans fat: In 2003 the FDA announced that trans fat was a contributing factor to coronary heart disease. If a product says it contains few or zero grams of trans fat, look at the nutrition label. Often it will be loaded with saturated fat, which can be just as unhealthful as trans fat. Example: One popular frozen snack makes the "zero trans fat" claim on the front of the label, but the nutrition facts panel shows it has 17 grams of saturated fat, 80 percent of the daily value of fat a person should consume.

Naturally fruit flavored: Some snacks display fresh fruit on the front label and state they are "naturally fruit flavored!" But often the real fruit contained in the package comes from a small amount of pear juice concentrate, a highly sugared form of fruit. Example: Betty Crocker Strawberry Splash Fruit Gushers are made primarily from pear concentrate and contain about 12 grams of added sugar. Also watch out for the label "made with real fruit." Most of these products have little nutrition as compared to their authentic fruit counterparts. Manufacturers put a drop of juice into the product, even though added sugar outweighs the fruit. When Ashley Koff Approved (AKA) was asked to "approve" a product developed by two moms that is USDA certified organic, AKA was appalled at the first three ingredients on the label—various forms of sugar and juice concentrate. A fruit snack? This was candy—albeit organic candy. Had they marketed it as such, AKA could have approved of these products for occasional consumption and with a portion control note. But as a fruit snack? That's absurd, organic or not.

> "Rich in calcium!" "Lower in sugar!" "High in vitamin C!" If it has to say it, it's likely not your best option. This is especially true about energy promises (or over-promises). Plain and simple, real food provides energy. It's just absurd that marketers promote their products with promises of more energy or better energy than food found in nature. After all, it isn't just the food's inherent energy but how the body uses it for energy that provides net energy results.

Contains antioxidants, contains vitamins, contains omega-3s: Sometimes foods and beverages are fortified with nutrients, such as "functional" soda pops or cereals with added vitamins and minerals. But fortifying a junk food does not undo its junkiness. Every year there is a new "it" ingredient among food manufacturers, which then gets media coverage. Soon after, we're looking for it in every food we eat. This poses nutrition issues as opposed to resolving them. First of all, a product with added nutrients from isolated forms is unlikely to benefit you the same way that those nutrients would when consumed in their natural form.

Second, it's possible to get too much of a single nutrient when it's added to a food product, and more isn't necessarily better.

The same holds true when it comes to the omega fatty acids. In the last 15 years or so we've been isolating a few omegas and concentrating them down to add to foods and supplements. But when you consider natural food sources that contain omegas, we often find a whole host of other healthy fats that we need but don't get when we consume isolated omega-3. Could we potentially see deficiencies of omega-5, -7, or -9 in the general population down the road if we continue to focus on supplementing omega-3 at a high dosage? Something to think about.

> **Profile Alert!** Did you see yourself as Profile 4 (The Chronic Dieter)? If so, pay attention to the following section.

DIET DETOX

We are what we eat. Though that statement is cliché, it's really true. If you performed a complete chemical analysis of your body, the report would list materials similar to those in foods: water, fat molecules, carbohydrates, protein complexes, and vitamins and minerals that help you to metabolize food and generate the energy you need to live. Think of the body as a self-maintaining factory; it is constantly regenerating itself down to every cell. Each month we renew our skin, every six weeks we have a new liver, and every three months we have new bones. To renew and rebuild these organs and tissues, we need to supply our bodies with the elements that have been lost as a result of constant use, degeneration, or aging. We also need to manage the imposters and substitutes that vandalize our normal functions. Let us explain.

In Dr. Mark Hyman's *UltraMetabolism: The Simple Plan for Automatic Weight Loss*, he calls for detoxifying the liver as a critical step to weight loss. His reasoning: a healthy functioning liver makes for a healthy functioning metabolism that can properly process foods.

He underscores the fact that toxins from both within our bodies and our environment can contribute to obesity. Hence, eliminating toxins and boosting your natural detoxification system is an essential component of long-term weight loss and a healthy metabolism.

Carrying excess fat isn't an issue of appearance per se. We know it plays a role in serious metabolic changes that interfere with the body's core systems and organs. Excess fat is a signal—an important one at that. It shouldn't be ignored.

We couldn't agree with him more. It's another vicious cycle that results in low energy: the more fat you have, the more toxins you retain, and the more toxins you retain, the harder it becomes to sustain a healthy metabolism to support ideal weight and energy production.

Too much fat can also slow down the time it takes for you to feel full, so you overconsume and fuel the cycle again. This is possible due to the hormones involved with fat metabolism. When faced with toxicity, our bodies respond by retaining water in an effort to dilute water-soluble toxins; our bodies also retain fat, to try and dilute fat-soluble toxins. Science has now proven that toxins in the blood can make a direct hit on our resting metabolic rates. Moreover, the same studies have determined that toxins affect the production of the thyroid hormones, which play a major role in your body's metabolism.

For 30 years now we've known that toxins can hinder our fat-burning engines by upward of 20 percent. Contrary to what you might think, fat cells are not inactive. Fat generates a multitude of biomolecules, including enzymes, hormones, and chemical messengers that tell our bodies what to do, which in turn affects how we look and feel. It has been said that our total body fat mass represents our largest endocrine (hormonal) organ since it is much larger than our pituitary, adrenal, thyroid, and sex glands.

Many of these molecules, such as estrogen, cortisol, and leptin, can promote more fat storage. The aromatase enzyme in fat, for example, converts testosterone into estrogen and further promotes fat storage. In fact, much of what fat does is continually signal the body to make more fat cells and store more energy via fat. In this process toxins are stored in fat as well, which aggravate the situation even more by promoting more fat storage. These toxins essentially mess with the proper signaling we need for maintaining a good ratio of fat to muscle.

Other factors can also contribute to the chaotic signaling. In our 24/7 lives where the lights are always on, we sleep rarely (and poorly), and we have an abundance of refined sugar available to keep us artificially charged, exacerbate the imbalance we experience in our body's internal workings. So again, it's a vicious cycle.

Toxins typically travel with the other impersonators found in our diets. Below is a list of common ingredients to avoid, followed by a few tips to cleaning up your environment. If you avoid these imposters, you'll automatically detoxify your kitchen and fuel your energy-producing power.

High-fructose corn syrup: It is NOT "just fruit plus corn." High-fructose corn syrup is a man-made ingredient that the body works harder to break down. When we eat this stuff, the result is digestive slowdown and increased risk of disease. Moreover, high-fructose corn syrup contains genetically modified (GMO) corn, so it's got unnatural ingredients in the corn that could create allergies and irritation, and have a negative impact on the body's energy. Stick to eating fruit and eating corn—your body gets them because they are real food. Watch out for high-*maltose* corn syrup too. As people begin to avoid high-fructose corn syrup, the food manufacturers are getting crafty with new variations on the same theme. Maltose is just another type of sugar that's often man-made. (For more about "real" versus "natural," see the box on page 80.)

Processed or added sugar: The sugar in a carrot is not the same as the sugar in a slice of carrot cake. The carrot has 30 calories and is loaded with beta-carotene, fiber, water, and potassium. The piece of cake is just a 300-calorie land mine of sugar and fat. It's the added sugars that are the problem in our diets today—not the natural sugar in foods untouched by man. Food manufacturers have used this added-sugar versus natural-sugar issue to their advantage, deceiving us into thinking their foods are made with real ingredients. Some have tried to pass high-fructose corn syrup off as natural, when in fact it's far from it. Others suggest that high-fructose corn syrup is fine in moderation, but the average American consumes 30 teaspoons of sugar daily—19 more teaspoons than advised by the World Health Organization. Clearly there is no moderation.

You can still go for sugar, even in excess once in a while, but do so knowingly (and use the cheat sheet in the box on page 80 as a guide). Everyone has a slightly different sensitivity to sugar. The more sensitive your moods and cravings are to sugar, the bigger bang for your buck you'll get by cutting back. So yes, you can have your cake and eat it too, but know that the effects of sugar in the system can last a few days. Highly processed, sugary items are the ultimate dead-battery food, such as regular ketchup, barbecue sauce, and peanut butter, for instance.

Keep organic fresh fruit and veggies cut up in the fridge; make smoothies using fresh fruits such as bananas, berries, and orange juice; or buy frozen, plain smoothie packs and then customize.

Artificial sweeteners (aspartame, saccharine, sucralose, acesulfame potassium, and cyclamate): These are hundreds to thousands of times sweeter than Mother Nature's sugar, and as such they can prevent you from feeling any sweet satisfaction from real food. If you get used to these little packets (or low-fat, sugar-free packaged goods that contain artificial sweeteners), suddenly fruit and sugar from our Mother doesn't taste so sweet. Studies prove that these sugars can trigger you to overeat. One Purdue study in particular found that even though these sweeteners don't contain calories, they cause weight gain in animals. The researchers speculate that the intense sweetness tricks the

Navigating the Sugar Minefield: Is it real or fake? A diamond or a cubic zirconia? Unfortunately, nutrition labels don't have to say where the sugar came from; they just have to provide total sugar content. To sleuth out the truth, read the ingredients list. All of the following are code words for added sugar:

Brown sugar	Fruit juice concentrates	Molasses
Corn sweetener	Glucose	Raw sugar
Corn syrup	High-fructose corn syrup	Rice syrup
Crystalline fructose	Honey	Sucrose
Dextrose	Invert sugar	Sugar
Evaporated cane juice	Malt syrup	Syrup
Fructose	Maltose	

Also, bear in mind that a food's contents must be listed on the label in descending order from most to least. The closer to the top of the list, the more of an ingredient is in the food. Aim to avoid or limit foods that contain any of the above-mentioned sugar aliases in the top three ingredients. If you focus on limiting the biggest offenders—soda, fruit drinks, candy, sweet baked goods, and ice cream—you'll do your body's energy metabolism well. More than 75 percent of our sugar comes from these items. Here's another way to look at it: if you eliminate just these five categories of foods from your diet for a year, you could save 78,000 calories and drop 20 pounds!

brain into thinking that calories are on their way when they aren't! The body gets confused, slows metabolism, and ramps up appetite. This imbalance in regulating calories leads to overeating. Also, artificial sweeteners are often found in combination with sugar alcohols such as maltitol, sorbitol, glycerol, and mannitol, among others. Sugar alcohols, which offer sweetness but do not get absorbed, are designed to replace table sugar. Because these molecules technically are not digested, they can linger in the digestive tract for a longer period of time and cause stomach upset in people with sensitive tummies or who consume excessive sugar alcohols.

Better alternatives: Use natural forms of sweetness such as organic honey, organic sugar, organic coconut palm sugar, maple syrup, molasses, and natural sweeteners such as organic stevia and erythritol in moderation.

Hydrogenated and partially-hydrogenated oils (ahem: trans fats): You know these clog your arteries already from all their media exposure, hence the halo over monounsaturated options such as extra-virgin olive oil. As we just noted, nature provides a balance of fats in many whole-food forms, so the key is to consume most of your fats in the whole-food form. When consuming products with fats in them, look to see if they contain a variety so you're not consuming just one type of saturated fat and zero monounsaturated fat. Limit your intake of the polyunsaturated from these vegetable oils (e.g., corn, sunflower, safflower, soy, and cottonseed), and use extra-virgin olive oil more often to replace these. Olive oil is heat-stable at low temperatures for cooking, which is the healthier way to cook anyway. Or, use other fats such as omega-3-rich chia and flaxseed oils, or blends such as an omega-3, -6, -9 mix or hempseed oil. As we'll see in Chapter 5, you'll want to eat more oily fish (salmon, sardines, herring, mackerel, and black cod) and use a variety of nuts and seeds such as walnuts, chia, hemp, and flaxseeds; as well as omega-3 fortified organic eggs to ensure you get sufficient omega-3 fatty acids for optimal health.

Enriched and bleached flour: After the refining process strips this flour of dozens of nutrients, it's then "enriched" through the addition of just four nutrients (B1, B2, niacin, and iron, in a synthetic form). Don't be fooled by the "enriched" name. You're not getting any richer. You're losing out on energy-fueling ingredients naturally found in these foods before man got a hold of them in the processing plant.

Monosodium glutamate (MSG): MSG should stand for "something that my body hates." Okay, maybe that's harsh, but for many people their reaction to it is just that—severe. For the rest, what we need to know is that MSG irritates our digestive tract, which is a big negative for optimal energy. For a list of MSG hideouts, see the following table.

MSG HIDEOUTS		
Foods always contain monosodium glutamate if any of these are in the ingredients list:		
Autolyzed plant protein	Glutamic acid	Sodium caseinate
Autolyzed yeast	Hydrolyzed plant protein	Textured protein
Calcium caseinate	Hydrolyzed vegetable protein	Yeast extract
Gelatin	Monopotassium glutamate	Yeast food or nutrient
Glutamate	Monosodium glutamate (MSG)	

Foods often contain MSG if any of these are in the ingredients list:		
Annatto	Flavoring seasonings (most assume this means salt and pepper or herbs and spices, which it sometimes is)	Protein-fortified anything
Barley malt	Flowing agents	Protein fortified milk
Bouillon	Gums	Rice or brown rice, syrup
Broth	Lipolyzed butter fat	Soy protein
Caramel flavoring (coloring)	Low or no fat items	Soy protein isolate or concentrate
Carrageenan	Malt extract or flavoring	Soy sauce or concentrate
Citric acid (when processed from corn)	Malted barley (flavor)	Soy sauce or extract
Corn syrup and corn syrup solids (partly depends upon process used)	Maltodextrin	Spice
Cornstarch	Milk powder	Stock
Dough conditioners	Modified food (or corn) starch	Ultra-pasteurized anything
Dry milk solids	Natural chicken	Vitamin enriched
Enriched	Pectin	Whey protein isolate

The mind, mouth, and reward system love the one-two salt-sugar punch. If we have salty food, do we crave sweet soon after? Often. So skip the soy sauce with sushi and perhaps an orange as dessert will satisfy you, versus needing ice cream or frozen yogurt.

A better alternative: Instead of using salt, season your meals with herbs, such as basil, oregano, and rosemary. These have anti-inflammatory properties, so they act like little energy optimizers in your body. Some ideas to have on hand in your kitchen:

- Fresh lemons

- Vinegar (balsamic, red-wine, apple-cider, etc.)

- Mustard

- Chiles

- Pepper

- Garlic

- Coarse sea salt or sesame salt

- A collection of fresh or dried herbs (e.g., basil, thyme, oregano, rosemary)

Look out for canned and packaged foods; they often contain way too much salt. Rather than using salt, cook with foods that naturally contain sodium, such as beets and their greens, kelp powder and other seaweeds, celery, chard, parsley, spinach, and kale.

Colorings known as red 3, yellow 6, blue 1, blue 2, and green 3:
Nature created colorful fruits and vegetables so they'd be attractive to us. They help with our hearts, our eyes, our skin, our digestive tract, and provide antioxidant benefits. The colors created in a lab with numbers on them are made to look pretty, but they are imposters and may exacerbate behavioral reactions in people with sensitivities. As this book was going to press, the FDA commenced an investigation into a potential link between food dyes and attention deficit hyperactivity disorder (ADHD) in children. Pretty soon, we could see these ingredients totally banned!

Salt: We all need a little salt (sodium) in our diets for the healthy function of nerves and muscles, including the heart. Salt is also essential for counteracting toxins in the body, for strengthening digestion, and for helping with the balance of acid-forming foods or acidic conditions created by nutritious foods such as beans, peas, grains, and meats. Although every cell in your body needs salt to work properly, we consume far more than we need. Your chance of being deficient is nil. That's why when we take in extra salt, we require extra water to reduce the sodium concentration to an optimal level, which results in excess water retention throughout the body that can tax our systems and drag our energy metabolism down. What's more, not all salt is created equal. Salts should have minerals, and they should be used in the cooking stage or ingredient combining—not as an additive and not as an extra preservative.

REDUCING ENERGY-DEPLETING TOXINS FROM NON-FOODS

It's not just about the foods that impart energy-depleting chemicals. Although it's impossible to avoid all the toxins in our world, there are a number of easy, practical things you can do to minimize your exposure. Some of them:

- Remove your shoes when entering your home, so you don't track germs and pollutants inside.

- Use air filters or commit to proper ventilation: HEPA/ULPA filters and ionizers can be helpful in reducing dust, molds, and airborne chemical compounds.

- Drink filtered water: use reverse osmosis systems or carbon filters. (Brita and Pur water systems allow you to fill up pitchers from your sink to filter and keep chilled in the fridge; you can also buy filters that go right onto your main tap in the kitchen.)

- Clean and monitor your heating system: this will reduce carbon-dioxide emissions that can literally poison you.

- Keep houseplants: live plants filter the air and add oxygen. Fill your home with spider plants, aloe vera, chrysanthemum, Gerber daisies, Boston fern, English ivy, and philodendrons.

- Purchase environmentally friendly cleaning products (baking soda and distilled vinegar products are relatively harmless).

- Avoid excess exposure to environmental petrochemicals, such as those found in gardening supplies, dry-cleaning fumes (air out your clothes when they come back from the cleaners), car exhaust, and secondhand smoke.

- Reduce or eliminate plastics, nonstick wares (i.e., Teflon-coated), and aluminums when you store (and, for that matter, cook) foods. Use nonplastic wares, containers, and wrappings, such as ceramic, porcelain, glass, and natural parchment paper.

- Use products with organic ingredients.

- Keep a tidy house (just the sight of a clean house can be energizing).

Don't look at this list and feel overwhelmed. You're not expected to change the way you live overnight. Just pick one thing to focus on for the week or month and then add more To Dos over time. Give yourself permission to modify your home and possessions in a relaxed and time-conscious manner.

I like to think of my body and my family's bodies
more scientifically when grocery shopping, and I don't pre-
pare meals with the thought that they're only pleasure feasts.
I prepare great-tasting gourmet meals for them with the
thought of refueling similar to a high-performance car: the
higher the octane (i.e., organic and local nonprocessed), the
more superior the output. I find when my kids eat balanced
nutritious meals, they listen better, play together better, and
are in better moods, which makes my energy level higher.

— D A N I E L L E   D I E T Z - L I V O L S I ,

founder and president of JagRma LLC (the NuttZo brand),
mom of 3, and grandmother of 13,
on secrets to energy success

PUTTING THE "OH" IN ORGANIC

It's got to be one of the top questions we get these days: do organic foods deserve a halo for goodness or a warning sign for hype?

First, the most important point to remember is that organic food means food. Period. Anything else is food plus chemicals. It provides us food sans the genetically modified seeds, without the use of pesticides, and with an optimal nutrient load (i.e., that which a plant or animal develops naturally). In that regard, it deserves more halos than many other halos dished out today in the food court, such as the terms *superfoods, all-natural*, and *healthy*.

In a general sense, eating organic food is more likely to satisfy you because it forces you to find foods close to Mother Nature. You're also likely to consume more plant-based nutrients that include phytochemicals for disease and wrinkle prevention, and to energize as nature intended.

But there's a caveat emptor to consider. While organic is healthier than chemically produced food, it cannot be the only deciding factor. Organic does not mean calorie appropriate, low sodium, low sugar, higher fiber, or nutrient balanced. You still have to evaluate organic products for these and other nutrition principles. Eating organic does not give you permission to ignore sensible portion control and achieving a balance of nutrients. So if you choose to have a helping of organic Oreos, for example (they do exist: "made from organic flour and sugar"), you still must take into consideration their fat and carbohydrate content and try to consume some healthy protein as well to get a better balance of nutrition.

Beware of Genetically Modified Foods

Nearly 60 percent of all manufactured food products in the United States today include soy—but not the soy you might affiliate with a healthy Asian diet or the natural bean, a sacred grain dating back thousands of years. Estimates suggest that 80 percent of the soy production in the United States is genetically modified. Initially, farmers planted GM soybeans in the weakened fields during crop rotations to rejuvenate the soil. Then they would discard the soybeans with the tilling of the field. But when the big business of today's commercial farming and food industries realized they could sell this mature crop rather than throw it away, they decided to find some uses for it. This move has created an industry worth billions, similar to that of the corn industry, which gives us high-fructose corn syrup.

Over half of the corn planted in the United States has been genetically modified using biotechnology, and the jury is still out on what this could mean for human health and the environment. We do know that one of the largest groups of diseases (autoimmune) as well as an exponential increase in emergency room visits for allergies all share a common theme: the body is intolerant to, irritated by, and being confused into attacking itself by something it's consistently exposed to. That GMOs permeate the list of foods and products (soy, corn, gluten) that are problematic for many people further helps connect the dots to the potential impact of GMOs. This seems to be enough evidence for at least 30 other countries to enforce significant restrictions or ban genetically modified versions of these foods entirely because they are not considered safe. In late 2010,

To keep abreast of all the latest science when it comes to food (and the chemistry of food), check out The Center for Science in the Public Interest (CSPI) at www.cspinet.org. The CSPI is a consumer advocacy organization whose twin missions are to conduct innovative research and advocacy programs in health and nutrition, and to provide consumers with current, useful information about their health and well-being. You can access reports and alerts, as well as stay current with what's going on at the federal level to ensure food education and safety.

Other resourceful organizations include the Non-GMO Project (www.nongmoproject.org), the Environmental Working Group (www.ewg.org), and the Organic Center (www.organic-center.org).

when the news hit about the genetically modified salmon we mentioned earlier—the one that grows twice the size in half the time—the war about how to label this "Frankenfood" began. Until we know more about how GM foods affect us and our energy metabolisms, we would do well to avoid or limit them and stick to the foods nature gave us. Because we don't know the long-term effect, or even short-term consequences, anyone consuming GMOs is, in effect, a guinea pig in a very large experiment.

MOM UP! JUMP-START YOUR TRANSFORMATION

It's really true: fast food is key to mom energy. And by that we mean food that's easy to assemble or prepare, that can be picked up or packaged for on-the-go, and that's above all, balanced. Traditional fast food that clogs our highway rest stops (and our arteries) is the true speed trap to our energy; it should be renamed "junk food." If you need to do just one thing differently this week, given all the information we've given you in this chapter, then let it be this: see if you can move one baby step away from relying on any speed trap set up by a fast-food chain or food manufacturer whose product reeks of ingredients that we've called out as those to avoid. Spend ten minutes checking out the labels in your pantry and refrigerator. Find at least three products you use consistently and find a healthier substitute for them. For example, replace your ketchup made with high-fructose corn syrup with one that's made with real tomatoes and organic sugar. Or swap out your peanut butter that contains added sugar for a jar of another made with just 100 percent nuts. The ingredients should say "100 percent peanuts" and nothing more.

CHAPTER 5

The Energy Exchange Part 2: Choose Energy Solutions in the Marketplace

Many people worry so much about managing their careers,
but rarely spend half that much energy managing their LIVES.
I want to make my life, not just my job, the best it can be.
The rest will work itself out.

— REESE WITHERSPOON

Clearly, avoiding the Frankenfoods and managing the marketing mayhem relies heavily on the choices made about what to eat (rather than what not to eat). All the tools our bodies need to function optimally and efficiently (read: produce and utilize energy) can be found in foods. We need food to live, to maintain the structure and function of our cells, and to support and fuel the systems that keep us going strong—immune, digestive, respiratory, circulatory, and so on. But some foods can have little to none of the nutrients we need, so when we eat nutrient-poor foods, we ask the body to work with fewer resources. When we provide nutrient-poor food *and* chemicals, then we ask the body to not only do its daily work with fewer resources, but we also ask it to combat additional challenges. We are starting to see research that indicates this may be a recipe for disease. Regardless, we know that it's a recipe for imbalanced energy, which tips our metaphorical scale in favor of burnout, premature fatigue, careless mistakes, and confusion. Put another way, when we perpetually consume nutrient-poor foods and beverages filled with harmful impersonators such as hydrogenated trans fats, saturated fats, and refined sugars—topped with preservatives, additives, and artificial flavors and colors—we set ourselves up for downgrading our energy metabolism and, in turn, our health.

The short answer to how this happens is that our bodies lose the capacity to self-heal efficiently as chronic inflammation takes over and our natural sources of "fixer uppers," such as antioxidants, get used up. In addition, without ample supplies nearby and continual replenishment of the nutrients we need to run our systems and natural defense mechanisms, the flames of aging, inflammation, and free-radical pandemonium hit high marks. And when the stress simmers over long periods of time—perhaps years—the entire waterfall effect among hormones, inflammatory chemicals, and free radicals sets the stage for accelerated aging. It also spells a recipe for energy disaster.

We know we're not the first to hawk the idea of everything in moderation, but it's really true that moderation is key to establishing a successful, energy-sustaining relationship with food and eating. We also understand the need for certain comfort foods and sugar on occasion; sometimes we give in to environmental cues that have us indulging in foods that provide more consolation than pure energy. By definition, comfort foods make us feel good, can lift a bad mood, and plain and simple be a form of stress relief. So in that regard sugar can be medicine, too! But there's a difference between a food that provides us immediate comfort and one that provides us lasting comfort. The secret is to combine sugar with other ingredients so it doesn't promote body chaos and send you through swinging highs and lows. If you eat sugar after a meal rich in lean proteins, healthy fats, and carbs, or eat sugar alongside these types of hormone-friendly foods, it won't incite such a huge insulin response as it would on its own.

If you haven't figured it out by now, we are complex beings. There is no magic pill, potion, or formula for guaranteed energy. So many things coalesce in our bodies to produce either the results we want or don't want. You've already gotten a good dose of information about diet choices, hormones, exercise, sleep, and so on. Plenty of scientific research exists about eating certain foods to support your health and energy metabolism, and learning how to balance others that don't necessarily maximize your energy goals. Don't panic: we won't ask you to do anything unrealistic, such as suddenly savoring wheat-grass juice. Our ideas are meant to resonate with your intuitive sense of how to care for yourself, which goes to the core of how you care about others. We're not here to act like overbearing mothers, forcing you to eat your vegetables, clean your plate, evict dessert from your life forever, and enter a zone of deprivation. Living a healthy, energetic life is much easier than that!

As with any healthy-eating guidelines, the goal here is to supply your cells and systems with the raw materials they need to function efficiently and optimally, inside and out. You don't want to give your body any excuse to downshift, so you need to be sure that at any given time it has all the resources it requires to stay alive and nourished to the max.

Before we even get to the details of filling a plate following the Mom Energy plan, though, let's take a quick detour to cover an area relevant to any woman searching for satisfaction in her diet: the food-mood connection.

THE FOOD-MOOD CONNECTION

It's easy to forget or ignore the difference between hunger and appetite. Each one of us is programmed to be hungry when our bodies need nutrients to survive; it's experienced as a drive to find food, and if we don't satisfy that need we'll feel an unpleasant sensation. Appetite, on the other hand, is more of a learned behavior; as the body's different senses trigger a desire for energy (i.e., food), even when we may not need it, over time we can respond to appetite cues that result in eating. This explains how one person can choose to eat poorly while another person chooses nutrient-rich foods when hunger strikes. Put another way, whereas hunger is a physiological need, appetite is a psychological desire. Anyone who has ignored hunger or overresponded to it knows what having an appetite out of control can be like. It's what leads to ingrained eating behaviors that lead to problems with weight.

We can't deny the emotional factor, which often provides the undercurrent to appetite. Our behavior around food is also intimately connected to deep emotional requirements such as the innate need to feel happy and satisfied. What we crave or use for comfort can be rooted in our eating patterns, which have profound psychological significance. This helps explain why you might go to the kitchen when you're unhappy, bored, stressed out, or sad and eat the leftover birthday cake rather than reaching for an apple. Likewise, when you're feeling insecure, you might eat a pastry mindlessly while on the phone with a friend. Or, as you say to yourself, "I am not going to feel sad; I am going to make the kids' lunches," you might then find yourself nibbling on the same treats you include in their bags as you assemble them. The other factor to consider is the circumstances—the context of the eating. You may be emotional, for instance, and then you enter the kitchen. The food is there and your mind goes to places that ultimately result in an override of your body's physiologic cues of true hunger, or lack thereof. Suddenly, your body's fullness gets rebooted and you find room for food no matter what.

Preventing a roller-coaster ride in your bloodstream that leads to a bona fide stress response is all about keeping those blood sugars balanced. This is accomplished by choosing carbohydrates that are filled with fiber, high-quality proteins, and healthy fats—all of which foster a slow and steady digestion. It's like the difference between driving a car in cruise control and putting your foot on and off the gas pedal to drive as fast as possible, dodging other cars and cops. When you set up your cruise control, you're effectively letting the car work the best it can—staying at a constant, doable speed and varying its speed appropriately as needed. The body, like your car, prefers the former approach—much less wear and tear. In doing so, you will be able to avoid those crazy, bingeing moments when you feel so out of control and live in constant reactive mode.

The fact that food can trigger your biological stress response system is significant. Numerous studies have shown that an overactive stress response is associated with overeating, changes in blood chemistry and hormones, and, in particular, a decrease in the amino acid tryptophan. Why is this important? This amino acid is a necessary building block in the mood-regulating neurotransmitter called serotonin. As you know, low levels of serotonin are linked to depression (or simply a depressed mood), insomnia, anxiety, anger, and continued bingeing on sugary, fatty foods. And what you may not know is that low serotonin levels are also associated with overeating, even bingeing, on carbohydrates because of its role in making tryptophan usable in the body as serotonin. All of which can then lead to energy loss and weight gain, especially the most unhealthy kind of all around the midlines and waistlines. Like a drug addict looking for our next hit, we want this serotonin when we attack the kitchen seeking sugary, nutrient-poor carbohydrates. Our brains release a short burst of serotonin when we eat simple sugars and carbohydrates; we feel good for a moment, but soon return to our low-serotonin state, and crash and burn. That's when we crave more sugar and carbohydrates in hopes of feeling that little high again . . . and the downward spiral continues.

Fat is another issue that helps us to prevent binges, and which stabilizes mood-energy. As we mentioned earlier, fat is not as stationary and inactive as a hibernating turtle. It can release hormones and chemical messengers that promote inflammation and will instruct your body to hold onto fat while breaking down components that are pivotal to energy metabolism, such as muscle. In 2005, researchers demonstrated that abdominal fat cells produce cortisol in large amounts. Japanese researchers have found that fat cells can generate free radicals that can then do damage throughout the body. They concluded that excess abdominal fat may bring on system-wide oxidative stress that has profound overall effects. So the lesson is clear: achieving and maintaining an ideal weight and a healthy muscle-to-fat ratio is important. It's also the cornerstone to optimal energy. The diet guidelines in this chapter will help you to accomplish this.

> **Profile Alert!** Once again, attention all Chronic Dieters (Profile 4). The following guidelines don't just speak to moms seeking to keep their energy reserves charged. These rules amount to a way of eating that will end all diets and help you to achieve the body—and constant energy levels—of your dreams.

BREAK THE RULE OF THE MEAL

Too often people get caught up in thinking that a snack is small and fun while a meal is large and happens at set times. But our bodies don't think this way. To employ the car analogy again, our bodies don't want to fill up with 1,800 calories in the morning and then allocate those calories throughout the day similar to how your car operates after you fill it up at the gas station. In fact, it won't know how to allocate all those calories at once, and it will shove a lot of them into fat storage. Your body much prefers to run like a racecar that has periodic pit stops about every three hours. How much we eat at that pit stop depends on a combination of our in-the-moment needs and the availability of food.

Although we will still use the word *meal* in this book, it helps to reconfigure your definition of this word to refer to it as an eating occasion. Forget the old rules of having to eat three meals and two snacks a day, or six small meals plus snacks. That's a pointless piece of advice. Every woman is different and should approach eating as would any other animal: she should eat when her body—and being—needs something. The caveats, of course, are what screw up many moms: (1) you have to recognize your body's internal hunger cues—tuning in to how you feel, what your food preferences are in the moment (and why), and what your goals are; and (2) you have to know how to make the most of those occasions and fill up on high-quality nutrients to satisfy all those needs. Many women fail to do this, resulting in endless grazing all day on mediocrity or storing up hunger and later pigging out on energy-depleting whatever.

Pit Stops versus Fill-ups. For optimal efficiency and to prevent fat storage, we need to refuel with only the amount of energy the body needs and will use about every three hours. Don't let yourself run on empty or backload—which refers to eating lightly all day and getting all your calories at night.

EAT ROUGHLY EVERY THREE HOURS

Less really is more in the energy equation. Give your body less and it will work more efficiently, producing higher energy. Put another way, in order to get the right amount of food without over-whelming the body and forcing it to store energy in the form of fat, you should aim to break up your eating into about three-hour incre-ments. Regular meals spaced about every three to four hours apart help keep the metabolism running in high gear. They also trigger the body to use good calories for fuel and give up the fat. This explains why someone who cuts back on overall calories may struggle to make excess fat go away. The body senses the reduction in calories, goes into survival mode, and holds tightly onto its fat. When food intake is spread throughout the day, however, this tells your body it's get-ting plenty of energy and can let go of that fat! Simply knowing that you get to eat again in a few hours has hidden benefits; you won't have that last-meal mentality that can lead you to overeat.

So aim to eat roughly every three hours no matter what, starting with a high-quality breakfast within an hour of rising. (Break the fast.) If you struggle with eating breakfast, then consider this: your body needs nutrients to turn it on—to shift from fat-storage mode to energy-using mode. The more you prolong this, the longer your body stays in fat-storage mode. Once you start eating correctly for optimizing your energy, you'll find that your body gets hungry approximately every three hours. You'll get into a rhythm of needing food consistently around that time frame. So even though it may feel strange at first, you'll eventually find yourself in a virtuous cycle of sustained energy.

How many of us have stuffed ourselves to the gills at a buffet-style Sunday brunch and felt lethargic (and guilty) the rest of the day? It sets the tone for the entire afternoon and pretty much disqualifies dinner because you just aren't in the mood or hungry enough. Similarly, we're all familiar with the uncomfortable sensation of being famished. The key to success is finding the middle ground between these two—not overdoing it to produce storage and not running on fumes. Just like when you try to find the balance between showering your kids with things they want and controlling how much you give them so they don't develop a sense of entitlement (not to mention a false sense of reality about money). Eating every three to four hours keeps the body on a relatively even keel. You'll avoid those energy highs and lows that spell metabolic disaster.

Remember, the body can only handle so much of any nutrients at one time, and if you don't need them for fuel (you may feel as if you're running a mom marathon in your mind but your body is not), then those excess calories will be stored as fat. Forcing your body to convert excess calories into fat puts a kink in its efficiency (hence the slow and sluggish feeling after a huge meal). Conversely, if you give your body less, you force it to use all that energy for fuel until you eat again, and you will feel the difference in sustained energy levels and mental clarity. Added bonus: you'll also produce less waste. That's the ultimate sign of an efficient body that makes use of all that you consume without needing to store extra fat. It's kind of like when you make a meal for the family and there's something that everyone likes. There are no leftovers, and cleanup is manageable.

No matter where I am or what I am doing, I have food supplies with me. Whether it be a banana or a Pure Bar, a Ziploc bag of Goldfish or a smoothie, I make sure I am providing my body with proper fuel throughout the day. My life is on the go all the time and sometimes sitting down for a full meal is not an option. But without food I am useless, so I make sure I always have my snacks so I am fueling my body no matter what I am doing.

— JESSICA MENDOZA,
professional softball player,
Women's Sports Foundation president,
and ESPN commentator

QUANTITY, QUALITY, AND BALANCE

Aside from feeding your body routinely, becoming a master at knowing what to eat and how much will take practice. Old rules need to be forgotten in this regard, too. You won't necessarily have to eat the same amount at every eating occasion. You might, for example, perform a hard workout on a Sunday afternoon but not feel the need for extra fuel to recover until Monday morning. Or you may be up with a sick child on a Tuesday night and feel like your eating is totally thrown off all day Wednesday. Choosing what to eat and when should be less about rules and more about tuning into what your body—and even your mood— needs. The way that nutrition has been taught historically and how it typically gets explained even today is counter to how the body works. It's not about calorie content, especially when it comes to energy. The body understands three ingredients:

carbs, protein, fat. Period. So yes, please stop counting calories and instead focus on getting the right balance of these three main ingredients to energy, and watch what happens. See if you can shift your focus from calories to nutrient balance. The ideas presented below will help you to do that. It's about becoming a "Qualitarian." This means, first and foremost, that you choose to be the gatekeeper for what goes into your body. That you don't feel deprived but rather empowered when you turn down a veggie burger with genetically engineered ingredients or hexane and enjoy one made from organic quinoa and mushrooms or a wild salmon burger. It also means saying no to a ready-to-eat salad of chemically sprayed lettuces in favor of cooking your own organic broccoli (great to start with frozen, too). And it means taking pride in listening to your own smarts instead of the front of a package or a commercial. Put simply, being a Qualitarian means choosing high-quality foods in the right portions to achieve a balanced meal that satisfies all your needs, from nutritional and physical to emotional. Whether you're a meat lover or a vegan, everyone can be a Qualitarian.

We all know that we need to manage our portions, and it does get confusing about what an ideal portion actually is, whether we're eating a piece of meat or diving into a bowl of gnocchi. But here's something to keep in mind when thinking about the relationship between eating and energy:

1 serving of carb, protein, or healthy fat = 1 hour of energy

So, if at each eating occasion you eat one serving of carbs, one serving of protein, and one serving of healthy fat, your body will have a total of three "power hours"—the first from the immediate energy of the carbs, and the second and third from the protein and fat, which take longer to break down.

Another way of looking at this math is to say that when you consume all of nature's foods—carbs, proteins, and fats—in respectable portions (which we'll get to shortly), you can maximize your energy metabolism over the course of three hours. You won't ever feel famished or stuffed, and your body will love it. Of all the guidelines in this chapter, this tenet—to achieve nutrient balance at every eating occasion—is most important.

General Guidelines

The overall principle of what to eat is simple: you choose one serving from each of the main categories—carbs, protein, and fat—and are allowed an unlimited amount of vegetables (no one is going to gorge on onions or spinach, so you get the point). For most people, this formula works, but there are lots of gray areas to consider. Some moms will have to bump their portions up to two servings of carbs and protein and one of healthy fat if they are exercising more or feeling the need for more. Any mother breastfeeding, for example, will need more carbs. If you're a vegan, you may end up higher on the carb side because your protein sources are often carb based. And some people may have two servings of protein with one carb and one fat because that balance helps their body address carb cravings and energy dips.

Already confused? Don't be intimidated here. Again, learning the ropes to finding your ideal serving of each category will take time and practice. These general guidelines are just that—general guidelines or guiding principles. They are not meant to be hard and fast rules, so don't look at this as a rigid list of exact measurements to be followed at all costs. You will need to improvise in some areas, as well as experiment with foods to address your personal choices and take into consideration social and cultural requirements. We cannot possibly give you a formula that works for every single situation or type of meal. You have to learn how to mix and match, and how to give and take. If you want to have dessert after dinner, but you also love the restaurant's breadbasket, then you may not want to order the lentil soup or hummus. Your carb box is already checked, so you just have to choose a healthy fat and protein for your entrée, and enjoy the vegetables. Use your common sense.

Never forgo carbs entirely at any given meal. One of the biggest mistakes you can make is to skip the carbs or save those carbs for a later feast. This will sabotage your energy equation. If you skip carbs at lunch thinking that you can then indulge in pizza with your kids at dinner, think again: you will more than likely be reaching for a carb-rich food by 3 P.M. to help you deal with the sugar craving you're sure to get. Remember to balance *all three nutrients* at every eating occasion no matter what. You really don't have any excuses to skip carbs given the volume of carb sources available today.

Remember, this is about choice! In fact, it's so much about choice that we encourage you to stop and ask yourself the following questions before you even decide what you're going to eat: *What am I looking for? What does my body crave? What does my inner voice say it wants?* Identify your body's chief needs first, and then decide what you're going to prepare for yourself (or purchase).

The following breakdown of foods in various categories will help you to choose wisely. Food is complex, so each food is listed by the dominant nutrient. Not every food you've ever heard of is on here, and the way in which the foods are listed doesn't mean you have to eat it exactly that way. You can steam or sauté your veggies, for instance. This breakdown is merely to help you begin to track how your meal is designed. Get creative about how you cook and prepare your meal with spices and seasonings. Note that there are two blended categories: one that includes foods that contain both carbs and protein, and another that has foods typically high in protein and fat.

Let us reiterate: don't panic about how to do the 1 + 1 + 1 with mixed categories. You'll get good at building your own eating occasions over time.

CARBS

Grains

Serving size: As indicated or your fist

amaranth; barley; bread, whole-grain, sprouted; buckwheat; bulgur (cracked wheat); crackers, whole-grain; kamut; millet; oatmeal, cooked (¾ cup); oats, whole (⅓ cup); pasta; pita, whole-wheat (½); quinoa; spelt; rice, basmati, brown, wild; teff; tortilla, corn, whole-grain, whole-wheat (½)

Fruit

Serving size: As indicated

apple (1 medium), apricots (3 medium), banana (½), blackberries (1 cup), blueberries (1 cup), cantaloupe (¾ cup), cherries (15), fresh figs (2), grapefruit (1 whole), grapes (15), mango (¾ cup), melon (¾ cup), nectarines (2 small), orange (1 large), papaya (¾ cup), peaches (2 small), pear (1 medium), pineapple (¾ cup), plums (2 small), raspberries (1½ cups), strawberries (1½ cups), tangerines (2 small)

Dairy/Dairy Replacements

Serving size: 6 ounces or as indicated

almond, rice, coconut, and soy milks, unsweetened, plain; coconut water, plain (11 oz); milk, organic; yogurt and kefir, plain, organic

Starchy Vegetables

Serving size: As indicated or your fist

beets; carrots (½ cup cooked or 2 medium raw or 12 baby); corn; peas; sweet potatoes or yams (½ medium baked); vegetable juices: carrot, beet, tomato (6 ounces); winter squash: acorn or butter nut

CARBS & PROTEIN

Beans/Bean-based Foods

Serving size: As indicated or your fist

beans: adzuki, black, cannelloni, edamame, garbanzo, kidney, lentil, lima, mung, navy, pinto, etc.; bean soups (¾ cup); bean dips (¼ cup); soy or veggie burger (4 ounces); tempeh (3 ounces); tofu (fresh: 8 ounces, cube: 3½ ounces)

Grains

Serving size: Your fist

quinoa

Dairy

Serving size: As indicated or your fist

cottage cheese, plain, organic; mozzarella, organic; ricotta, organic; yogurt, plain, Greek, organic (6 ounces)

PROTEIN

Meat, Fish, Poultry & Eggs

Serving size: As indicated or palm of your hand

beef, lean cuts; bison, buffalo, and other game; chicken, breast only; Cornish hen, breast only; eggs (1 whole or 3 egg whites); egg substitute (⅔ cup); fish; lamb, leg; shellfish (3 ounce fresh or ¾ cup canned in water); turkey

FAT & PROTEIN

Nuts & Seeds

Serving size: As indicated

almonds, brazil nuts, cashews, and hazelnuts (10 to 12); peanuts (18); hemp seeds, pistachios, pine nuts, pumpkin seeds, sesame seeds, sunflower seeds (2 tablespoons); nut butters (1 tablespoon)

Dairy

Serving size: 1 ounce

fattier cheeses: blue, Brie, Camembert, cheddar, Colby, Comte, Gorgonzola, gouda, Gruyère, Havarti, Manchego, Monterey Jack, Muenster, provolone, Swiss

FAT

Oils

Serving size: 1 tablespoon

canola, chia, coconut, extra-virgin olive, flax, grapeseed, hemp, olive, sesame, walnut

Nuts & Seeds

Serving size: As indicated

chia seeds (1 tablespoon); macadamia nuts (10); pistachios (¼ cup); walnut and pecan halves (7 to 10)

FAT (continued)

Fruit

Serving size: As indicated

avocado (¼ cup); coconut, shredded, unsweetened (3 tablespoons); olives (8 to 10)

Spreads

Serving size: 1 tablespoon

cream cheese, low-fat, plain; Neufchâtel; pesto; tapenade

NON-STARCHY VEGETABLES

Serving size: Unlimited

artichokes, arugula, asparagus, bamboo shoots, bean sprouts, bell or other peppers, bok choy, broccoli, broccoflower, Brussels sprouts, cabbage (all types), cauliflower, celery, chicory, chives, collard greens, cucumber/dill pickles, eggplant, escarole, garlic, green beans, kale, leeks, lettuces, mushrooms, okra, onion, radicchio, radishes, salsa (sugar free), sea vegetables (kelp, etc.), snow peas, spinach, sprouts, squash (yellow, summer, or spaghetti), Swiss chard, tomatoes, water chestnuts, watercress, zucchini (Italian)

When choosing animal and animal products, choose organic. For fish, there isn't a definition for "organic" so choose sustainable seafood, which includes most wild fish and some select farm-raised seafood.
(For help, visit www.seafoodwatch.org.)

Try Tracking

Now that you know the general formula for your eating occasions, it helps to track what you eat every day for the first week so you can really see how much you're eating from each category and whether or not you're truly getting a good balance. At the end of each day, ask yourself two questions: (1) Did I eat about every three hours? If not, why not? (2) How many servings of carbs did I have at each eating occasion? This is how you may find out that gosh, your breakfast contained six servings of carbs and then you had zero carbs until dinnertime, at which point you gorged on seven servings of them.

If you reduce your portion sizes and still find yourself very hungry, then you've got three options to consider:

- Choose higher fiber foods.

- Eat more veggies.

- Check in with yourself to see if you're actually not hungry, but not stuffed. Many people become so conditioned to big feelings of fullness that they have to reacquaint their bodies to feeling like they've had just enough and will be okay for another couple of hours before they eat again. Remember: your body works best when it's underwhelmed.

Don't let yourself get too hungry. Blood-sugar drops are exhausting and emotionally straining (for your kids too!). I always carry a bag of energy with me that includes a healthy, balanced snack that doesn't skimp on protein. I love my nuts and seeds.

— MYRA GOODMAN,
co-founder of Earthbound Farm,
cookbook author, and mom

Due to the attention on carbs over the past decade, many of us have gotten pretty good at knowing the difference between a "good carb" such as whole-grain bread and a "bad" one such as plain white bread stripped of its nutrients and fiber. But all the focus on carbohydrates has left people still confused about proteins and fats. And there's a lot that can be said about these two critical macronutrients our bodies need to create sustained energy. Let's take a look at each of these in turn, followed by some general guidelines for making the most of your eating experience.

Choose an Assortment of Proteins

Proteins are found in both animal and vegetable sources. However, each food source contains differing varieties and amounts of amino acids, which are the individual chemical units that comprise proteins. In other words, amino acids are the building blocks of proteins. The terms *complete protein* or *high-quality protein* are used to refer to those proteins that provide all of the essential amino acids in a proportion needed by the human body. A couple of the essential amino acids play a critical role in feeding the mitochondria, which, you'll recall, are the energy units of cells.

Proteins play an important role in our body. The most well-known is their role in building lean body mass (muscle), but many proteins are also enzymes which mean they are messengers in cellular communication that signal metabolism and immune responses among other core functions. When consumed, your body goes to work breaking down proteins into their amino acids, which then get absorbed and transported by the blood to cells for use. The mere act of breaking down protein burns calories and keeps your blood sugar stabilized. Amino acids can then be converted to glucose and used as energy, or they can form new protein molecules needed by the body.

While the body needs protein daily, it can get too much. The body does not store excess protein and the process for removal requires the liver and kidneys to work hard at removing these larger molecules. These organs are adept at doing so, but if it becomes a longstanding pattern or if they are in a weakened state, this can prove challenging to them and they may signal their displeasure by working less effectively or even going on strike. They can also lose their functionality if the body doesn't get sufficient carbs, in which case it uses protein for energy but creates significant waste.

The word *protein* gets thrown around a lot today. One reason for this is because there are so many sources of protein available now including those from animals and other vegetarian options such as whole grains, beans, nuts, and seeds. But a key energy distinction lies in whether the protein is isolated—which means extracted from the whole food through some processing—or if it remains in the whole-food form. This can make a big difference in nutrient quality and digestibility. When it comes to soy protein, which shows up in so many places such as powders, bars, and shakes, be aware that soy protein isolate can be problematic for some people. This form of soy is produced by removing nutrients from the whole soybean, which may play a role in modifying the hormonal effects of soy—raising concerns for people with thyroid imbalances, certain cancers, and metabolic syndromes like polycystic ovarian syndrome.

Vegetarian sources of protein offer tremendous nutritional profiles, but vegetarian doesn't always mean healthy. There are poor-quality vegetarian proteins sold on the market that can be as energy-sapping as low-quality animal protein.

As already mentioned, wherever possible, seek organic sources of protein, especially from animals (including whey and egg white) and soybeans. This means that no chemicals were given to the animals or sprayed on the plants, and that no genetically modified seeds were used. The choice between animal and vegetable sources of protein should be one of personal preference, ethics, environmental concerns, and taste. We say this because it is a myth that vegetarians and vegans can't get sufficient protein from a plant-based diet. Yes, some plants have components that can block absorption of some proteins, but that doesn't mean one cannot achieve adequate protein intake. It merely means that it requires knowledge and planning.

When it comes to vegetarian sources of protein, try hemp protein (e.g., powder, seeds) for its nutrition profile and ease of digestibility; and several of the pea/quinoa/rice blends are satisfying, healthy options. Quinoa and hemp are naturally complete proteins whereas the others are not, so you would need to consume other sources of amino acids throughout the day to arrive at a more complete profile. A note on hemp: it's made from the seeds of the hemp plant and thus it does not contain THC, the psychoactive component of the marijuana plant. If you feel really good from eating hemp, it's coming from true energy and nutrition and not a drug (this includes the healthy fat source GLA, present only in hemp). Another item to note is that some products will contain sprouted quinoa, grains, nuts, or seeds. Sprouting is an excellent way to improve the availability of the protein; these are great for those with digestive issues where absorption may already be challenged.

ASHLEY'S ENERGY ADVICE:

I get asked all the time about energy bars and shakes. Are they a smart choice? Are they Ashley Koff Approved? Sometimes. But proceed with caution. Many people just grab a bar or whip up a protein shake after dinner. Or they will have two or three during the day because the small size of the bar means they don't register the caloric density they've consumed (some bars can have as many calories and be as nutrient poor as a Caesar salad or slice of pizza), wondering why they find weight loss or maintenance such a challenge.

Two general nutrition concerns apply strongly to the category of ready-made bars and shakes: unnecessary processing and unnecessary use of preserving agents. For example, if you're consuming a bar with nuts and dried fruit, why not just choose an apple with some nuts or nut butter instead? The difference in calories and nutrient balance can be significant. For starters, many bars' carbohydrate content is too much (two to four servings) while its protein content is minimal—not even one serving. Many bars are high on the glycemic index, meaning they will stir a spike in blood sugar, and this is often due to lots of dried fruit—not necessarily added sugar. They often don't give you enough to eat from a practical standpoint. You eat three to five bites quickly and don't register a full signal, so you seek something else to satisfy you, which can then throw your nutrient load overboard. Also, many of these items contain nonorganic versions of fruit that should only be eaten from organic sources. They further may contain processed or chemical ingredients and isolated soy protein (remember: if eating soy, eat the whole non-GMO bean to get the protein, fiber, and healthy fats). The excuse of "a bar is for convenience" has gone too far. How inconvenient is an apple and some nuts? This is what many bars purport to be, but then again, you get fiber and water and phyto-nutrients from the skin of the apple, which you probably won't get in the bar.

Know the distinction between a desire for a bar or shake versus the true need for convenience. Can you take a little extra time and assemble something yourself? If not—and keep in mind I'm a realist who gets how life can demand some quick fixes—make sure to choose a product that doesn't have you trading convenience for optimal health. Look for extra sugar and salt. Count the grams of carbohydrates, proteins, and fats.

Indeed, there is a time and place for bars (e.g., traveling, post-gym, a back-up plan for emergencies), but the whole-food route is always a better option when it's available. And finally, it's important to consider what else is in there aside from artificial ingredients. In an effort to make protein bars, shakes, and powders as powerful—and marketable—as possible, as well as to differentiate their brand, manufacturers routinely add herbs, vitamins, minerals, and other nutrients. As such, a final consideration should be a review of these ingredients, an assessment of their quality, an assessment of any possible contraindications with medications, sleep patterns (if you are having a protein drink or bar at night that has stimulating ingredients it could keep you awake), and individual sensitivities. For example, I recently couldn't figure out why I was having shaky hands and my pulse was racing. Then I realized I had been sampling a sport protein powder for work and it was giving me the same issues that I have with caffeine. The culprit? An intended energizing combo of maca root and other potent stimulant herbs!

Boost Your Brain with Balanced Fat

High-fat fish such as salmon are called brain food for a reason. Fats don't just add cushion and warmth; they are necessary for energy production, and even for your sanity. About two-thirds of our brains are composed of fat, and the protective sheath around communicating neurons is 70 percent fat. So in a sense we need fat to think and to maintain healthy brain function, which in turn help us to feel balanced; in particular, the class of essential fatty acids called the omega-3s and omega-6s play a crucial role in brain function as well as normal growth and development.

> Ever heard of mommy brain? Feel that your memory was sharper before kid number one and is gone after number three? There's some nutritional rationale for this, which goes back to the idea that when pregnant, the body preferentially gives our DHA over to the baby to support its brain development. So if we don't replenish, we net at a loss. Since DHA intake doesn't appear to save us in the late stage (once we have dementia, or worse, a cognitive disease such as Alzheimer's), what we do know is that we have to restock our stores all along the way.

The omega-3 fats in salmon as well as other cold-water fish, nuts, seeds, algae, and soybeans have numerous proven health benefits, including those that protect the heart. One omega-3 in particular, docosahexaenoic acid (DHA), is the nervous system's favorite fat. It's the most abundant omega-3 fatty acid in the brain and the retina of the eye. A full 50 percent of the weight of your neurons' plasma membranes are composed of

DHA. Low levels of DHA or a deficiency results in reduction in logical thinking, hormonal changes, poor memory, mental decline, a higher rate of cell death among brain cells, depression, and an increased risk for heart disease. DHA not only provides structure to neurotransmitters and facilitates neurotransmitter activity, but it also increases neurotransmitter receptor density, which allows the brain to make use of serotonin and dopamine signals (good for good moods!). Because of DHA's effects on brain and eye development, many prenatal vitamins for women now include DHA supplements. DHA protects the brain and acts as an anti-inflammatory.

Healthy essential fats such as DHA are at an all-time low in moms' diets, whereas unhealthy fats (e.g., saturated and trans), are at an all-time high. But it's healthy fats that help fat-soluble vitamins such as A, D, E, and K move around the body; create sex hormones; build cell membranes; lower LDL (bad) cholesterol while raising HDL (good) cholesterol; and contribute to the health of skin, eyes, nails, and hair.

In the omega-6 family, gamma-linolenic acid (also known as GLA) is one of the all-stars. Well known as a stress-reducing nutrient, GLA is largely deficient in the standard American diet because it's a rarer oil, found in seed oils such as borage oil, evening primrose oil, black currant oil, and hemp oil.

People are more likely to overdo other omega-6s from sources such as refined vegetable oils, which can increase—not decrease—inflammation. Soybean oil, much of which hails from GMO soybeans, for example, is ubiquitous in fast foods and processed foods; in fact, 20 percent of the calories in the American diet are estimated to come from this single source. This can create an imbalance of too many omega-6s and not enough omega-3s, which is partly being blamed for the rise of myriad diseases from asthma and heart disease to many forms of cancer and autoimmune diseases. The imbalance also may contribute to obesity, depression, dyslexia, and hyperactivity. One study showed that violence in a British prison dropped by 37 percent after omega-3 oils and vitamins were added to the prisoners' diets!

The omegas don't end there. We can't forget about the omega-9s, -5s, and -7s (do you feel as if you're playing cards yet?). Technically, olive oil is an omega-9. Omega-7, known as palmitoleic acid, may appear to have minor status in the world of monounsaturated fats but its health benefits are hardly such. Omega-7 helps regulate fat and blood sugar metabolism (in adipose tissue and in the pancreas). In vitro studies suggest that omega-7 helps improve the function of the insulin-producing beta cells of the pancreas. And when it comes to the skin, omega-7 is no minor leaguer—it's a major fatty acid in epithelial cell membranes. This means skin, blood vessels, and mucous membranes. The presence of omega-7 in the epithelial cell membrane plays a protective role including inhibiting bacterial growth, as well promoting tissue recovery and healing. Research specifically on sea buckthorn oil (which contains 30 to 40 percent omega-7), shows its role in improving eczema, acne, oral and stomach ulcers, and vaginal irritation/dryness. Common dietary sources of omega-7 fatty acids include wild salmon, macadamia nuts, and sea buckthorn berries.

Omega-5, otherwise known as myristoleic acid, is less common in nature—found primarily in the seed oil from plants in the Myristicaceae genus where nutmeg is the most well known; the oil is also extracted from saw palmetto. Myristoleic acid extracted from saw palmetto has been shown to effectively combat cancer cells in prostate and pancreatic cancers. Additionally, omega-5 may play a key role in the inhibition of 5-lipoxygenase, a mediator of inflammation, thus, by acting in this anti-inflammatory capacity it helps to promote appropriate inflammation in the body. Food sources of omega-5, beyond extracting myristoleic acid from the aforementioned plants, include the fat of marine animals (wild Alaskan salmon), beavers, and bovines.

Getting a good balance of these fats is pretty easy. One key takeaway from this omega story is that rather than picking one or two favorites, which Mother Nature doesn't do, think of your omega consumption as an orchestra—all the different omegas playing together make the sweetest music. Whether food or supplement, consider making the choice that provides an array of omega fatty acids. After all, a whole-food approach to nutrition will help ensure you get omega-5, -7 and -3, -6, -9 for optimal health.

As we've already noted, simply reduce your consumption of processed and chemically laden foods; also reduce the use and consumption of polyunsaturated vegetable oils (e.g., corn, sunflower, safflower, soy, and cottonseed). Switch to extra-virgin olive oil as much as possible (it's heat-stable so use it to cook, too). Eat more oily fish (salmon, sardines, herring, mackerel, and black cod) as well as walnuts, flaxseeds, and omega-3 fortified eggs. Consider supplementing with a true fish oil like one from wild salmon, which will deliver all the omegas found in this fish naturally.

NINE WAYS TO PRACTICE A HEALTHY EATING ROUTINE

Below is a collection of ideas to help you maximize the execution of the ideas described in this chapter. See if you can begin to fold these simple ideas and, in some cases, actionable steps into your life.

Watch Out for "Energy" Bars Marketed as Low Sugar or Low Carb

The vast majority of these "diet-friendly" bars contain preservatives and modified ingredients such as sugar alcohols. Sugar alcohols, which we mentioned earlier, are designed to offer a low-carb sugar profile and can present a challenge to the digestive system; they are not meant to be absorbed and as such often cause gas and irritation. So instead of helping your energy level, these sugar alcohols and other preservatives may further irritate your entire system and, put simply, clog your energy flow. Opt instead for soybean in the whole-food form (edamame, tofu, etc.) versus bars and other food products made with isolated soy protein. There are great nutrients in the whole bean, fiber, and omega-3 fatty acids, among others that are lost when the protein is isolated.

Remember, carbohydrates are what the body needs for energy. Ingredients that impersonate carbs for taste but don't provide genuine energy are cheating the body, and the body always catches on to cheats—often resulting in an irritated digestive system.

Stock Your Freezer

With the economy, food-safety issues, and time efficiency on everyone's mind, the freezer offers one of our best tools for nutrition for optimal health. Whether it's fruits, vegetables, or fish, these foods are frozen immediately after they are plucked from a tree or the sea and washed. This means that these foods are literally frozen in time at their peak freshness and don't endure as much exposure to potential contaminants. What's more, stocking your freezer means you always have a healthy option available. With a quick run under hot water or a steam, you can create a truly fresh dish in minutes. What's more, frozen goods last a long time so you get your money's worth. Here are some tips to help you be freezer savvy.

- Buy frozen organic fruits and vegetables, especially when it comes to berries and other fruits that go bad quickly when you buy them fresh. You can use organic frozen berries in yogurts, on top of frozen desserts, or in a smoothie in lieu of ice. When buying frozen vegetables, you can defrost them in the refrigerator overnight and use them the next day. Or place them in the fridge in the morning, and they'll be ready to cook when you arrive home in the evening.

- Order takeout or buy prepared food that can be tweaked at home in seconds for a blast of nutrition. Always have frozen veggies on hand to add to dishes. Spinach, broccoli, and soybeans can be added as a side dish or thrown into pasta sauces and on top of frozen pizzas. Add extra veggies to a dish of beef and broccoli from the Chinese restaurant (ever notice there's way more beef than broccoli in those containers?); correct the imbalance with your own assortment of veggies and extend the dish from four to eight servings.

- Frozen wild or quality farmed fish is another example of better quality and freshness. Pull frozen fish from the freezer and place it in a bowl to defrost in the fridge. When you start to prepare dinner, mix thawed veggies with the fish, place them in a saucepan, and pour vegetable broth (low-sodium please) and spices into the saucepan. Cover and boil or steam for five to seven minutes. Voilà!

- Store individually wrapped, single-serving portions of meat, poultry, and fish in the freezer.

Engage Your Young Kids

Food education starts early. Challenge young kids to weekly contests by asking them to count how many (natural) colors are in the fridge and the freezer. Take them with you to the grocery store once in a while to show them how you shop and why you're choosing one item over another. Kids will appreciate learning about food and its nutritional value. Contrary to what you might think, they don't necessarily want junk food all the time.

The following is a list of top fish to buy,
many of which are rich in healthy fats that you
won't find in other foods to the same degree.
Unless otherwise noted, aim for wild-caught,
sustainably sourced varieties:

Abalone (U.S. farmed)	Herring	Salmon (from Alaska or British Columbia)
Anchovy	Hoki	Sardines
Bigeye (troll or pole caught)	Mackerel	Squid (from California)
Black cod	Mussels (farmed)	White sea bass
Catfish (U.S. farmed)	Oysters (farmed)	Tilapia (U.S. farmed)
Clams (farmed)	Rainbow trout (U.S. farmed)	Tuna (troll or pole caught albacore and yellowfin)
Dungeness crab	Rock lobster	
Halibut	Sablefish (from Alaska or British Columbia)	

For more information about
these fish and others not listed, check out the
Monterey Bay Aquarium's Seafood Watch website
at www.seafoodwatch.org.

Keep It Safe, Keep It Simple

The kitchen should be a safe zone. Don't keep too many treats lying around or they will get eaten (sooner than you think). You should go out for treats. Think of it this way: if your excuse is "Oh,

I had the cookies in the house for the kids," and you find your-self consuming them, then you've just let your kids enable your dysenergy.

Also keep it simple. Don't become a short-order chef. Kids need to learn how to eat like adults so you don't spend hours in the kitchen fixing food that fits each member of the household's palate. If you allow this then you must really like your kitchen. Getting your kids to try all kinds of food makes it easy to pre-pare a regular dinner that everyone enjoys. And by all kinds of food, we're also talking about how it's prepared. Take chicken, for example, and do it every way possible—grilled, broiled, and roasted. We all know we (moms and kids!) need to eat more veg-gies. Choose two or three per night and try roasting or baking your veggies rather than plain old steaming them. Don't forget that kids love to dip so let them do so with pasta sauce, hummus, or aged balsamic vinegar with a drizzle of olive oil.

Examples of staples to keep around: organic milk, brown rice, organic eggs, whole-grain bread, apples, strawberries, organic cheese, black beans, extra-virgin olive oil, crushed garlic, veggie or chicken broth, frozen organic vegetables (e.g., spinach, soy-beans, broccoli, asparagus), organic chicken breasts and fish in your freezer, and tomatoes. You can whip up several dishes using these basics.

Clean Out Your Kitchen Closets

Pantries are overrated. They just encourage you to buy more food that you don't need. And why would you want to have food that keeps for months? That only means it is full of preservatives, additives, and chemicals that you don't want anyway.

Once a season, go through your cupboards (and your refrig-erator while you're at it) and check expiration dates. Just as you would revamp your clothing closets at the beginning of each season, do the same for your kitchen. If it's been there since last month (or maybe even last year!), and you haven't eaten it or used it in a recipe, it's time to go. You can do a cupboard exchange with friends—asking them what their secrets are. Ask to take a look in your friends' cupboards and refrigerators to see if they have ideas you can use, too.

Some of our pantry staples: whole-wheat flours, organic white and brown sugar, pure maple syrup, organic hulless popcorn, steel-cut oats, whole-wheat pasta, black beans, kidney beans, garbanzo beans, brown rice, pasta sauce, tomato paste, low-sodium soups and broths, cacao, nuts and seeds, oils, dried fruit, and spices.

Don't Be Fooled

Navigating the supermarket today can be tricky. Supermarkets now place junk food next to healthy food. They also make it easy to grab what they want you to grab by how they place goods and attract your attention through specials and signs. Here's a classic example: you're in the produce department and next to the organic greens is a line of salad dressings. Next to the heads of broccoli is a sauce that can be used when cooking the veggies. But if you were to make an effort to peruse the aisle dedicated to sauces and dressings, you'd be able to find a much better one than those tossed randomly in the produce department. Avoid the samples handed out unless they are of something you love but don't want to have at home. Don't rely on the person doing the demonstration—they mean well, but may not point out any downsides to the product ingredients. Read the label yourself.

Be Careful about Buying in Bulk

Buying in bulk often does not save you money. If you don't read the expiration date and purchase items that expire very soon (and you don't have a family of 15), then it's wasted money. Bear in mind too that if the bulk product was in a bin and is a food that is sensitive to oxygen and light (e.g., nuts, seeds, grains), then you're doing yourself no favors. Most bulk foods come with preservatives and additives—it's what allows it to be sold in bulk! That said, load up on organic frozen fruits and vegetables that your local big-box store sells. Buying in bulk can help you get organic at lower cost. You can also visit company websites to learn new ways to use ingredients you buy in bulk so that you use up the product before the expiration date and get your money's worth.

Health is within everyone's budget. The goal is to realize true savings and avoid buying tons of items no one in the family enjoys (and refuses to eat). Nothing has been saved if no one is happy.

The True Power Lunch

Eating a nutrient-balanced lunch can do more for your P.M. energy than just a high-carb or high-protein one can. Remember, when we get a balance of nutrients and keep it to about one serving of each (carb plus protein plus healthy fat) plus unlimited vegetables, the body gets three power hours. For extra energy, take a B vitamin complex or your multivitamin/mineral supplement with your lunch. It will optimize the metabolism of your food for energy.

Allocate Your Alcohol

You can still have your wine and drink it, too. But be mindful of how much you are consuming. A drink while you cook, then another glass or two at dinner can amount to too much. It will disrupt your sleep cycles and potentially disturb your digestion as well. For most women, one five-ounce glass is plenty. Savor it with your meal and drink sparkling water with a wedge of lemon or orange while you cook.

Is white wine as good as red? There's been a lot of media frenzy over red wine's super-antioxidant resveratrol, but what about whites? According to Drs. Dipak Das and Alberto Bertelli of Connecticut and Milan respectively, white wine derives its cardio-boosting effects from two antioxidants—tyrosol and hydroxytyrosol—which are also found in olive oil. Interestingly, these antioxidants, such as resveratrol, trigger a gene that may slow aging, and have benefits for diabetes prevention and kidney function. So go on, love your whites as much as your reds. If you're like Kim Basinger, you'll take white wine and cut it with sparkling water. To really reduce the amount of sugar (and calories) you're consuming, opt for a dirty martini. Stay away from soda and fruity or creamy drinks. And when you do indulge, count your drink like it's a dessert instead of just a beverage.

THE ENERGY EXCHANGE

Remember, even though you now have all this information about what to eat and what not to eat, healing energy issues is not about displacing or replacing food and beverage consumption with other excesses, such as shopping, over-exercising, drinking too much alcohol, etc. Many women try to mask their symptoms of low energy with something that makes them feel invigorated, albeit superficially. You can spend a small fortune at the mall, for instance, but that doesn't really do anything for you but drain your bank account and your energy due to the stress of going broke. We've met moms who admit they've overspent money on superfluous items because they didn't want to face reality and get to the bottom of why they were sad. So they not only max out their credit cards, but they go home still longing to feel better as they juggle demanding children. The kitchen then calls to them, and they start eating—chips, a carton of ice cream, and liter of soda for the caffeine—and then they usually end up feeling bad about all those calories and money spent. The next day, their physical and emotional energy is really low, and the cycle can repeat itself. And if it's not the mall calling them, it could be the cocktail bar, or engaging in fantasies of living an easier life—or even cheating on a partner to get energy from the excitement of an affair. There's definitely something to be said for the energy derived from behaviors that have a "forbidden" factor or "forget it for a moment" component.

The takeaway here is you don't want to eat around a craving or exchange one energy drain for another. Doing so is called "eating transference," meaning that you go shopping, for example, instead of eating—in essence, you binge at the mall. Or maybe you're the type to use excessive exercise as a way to avoid eating. The human body is smarter than you think. You'll manage to avoid eating what you really want but pay consequences later in other terms. Another example: if you want chocolate but have a salad, lean protein, tea, and berries because your mind tells you that's better, chances are later on you'll have the chocolate anyway, but likely devour it on a greater scale than if you had just chosen chocolate with tea the first time around.

In all of these scenarios, what you're really aching for is permission to just cry, scream, or do *anything* that will take you out of the current moment. The lesson here is clear: even though certain foods and actions can change your spirits or help you forget your stress, these are often Band-Aids at best and energy zappers at worst. In later chapters, we'll provide ideas to help you find other ways to lift your spirits, overcome those emotional low notes, and keep your emotional baggage in check. For now, we just want you to be aware of this all-too-common cycle. Learn to spot it when it begins to surface. Energy will travel wherever you decide to take it.

Aim to live by the four tenets: quality, quantity, frequency, and balance. Start slowly. This week, try structuring one eating occasion each day by our balanced 1 + 1 + 1 formula. See how that one tiny shift makes all the energetic difference by the end of the week.

PART III

REHABILITATE

CHAPTER 6

Rehabilitate Your Body: Relieve Advanced Imbalances

It doesn't get any easier, it just gets different.
You respond differently.
You have different needs.

— LISA MARIE PRESLEY
on motherhood with different-aged kids

Congratulations. You've begun to take control of your health. You've started to master the art of choosing the right foods for you and your family. You've taken a few steps to reorganize your life and the foods you bring into your home. Hopefully you've noticed an uptick in the level of your everyday energy. Your stress is reduced. Your body is feeling better. And your mood is happier. Maybe your family members have noticed a difference too (or just a few changes in the kitchen!). But the shifts you need to make don't end there. It's possible that you are still fighting other problems that could be getting in the way of true success. We face the possibility of a lot of additional health concerns that make it nearly impossible to balance our energy equations just by focusing on how we spend our time and what we put into our bodies.

So now we turn to the second part of this book where we look at ways in which we can rehabilitate the body—getting it back to a fully charged state. For some of us, trouble comes from a chronic medical condition that requires routine maintenance, such as irritable bowel or diabetes, while for others it stems from a temporary blip in life such as menopause or an underactive thyroid that needs treatment. In this chapter, we're going to take you on a tour of some of the most common health conditions that will sap any mother's energy, and what you can do about them. Then, in the next chapter, we'll cover when and how to embark on a detox regimen, as well as give guidance on supplementing. Sometimes, we just need to hit "reboot" and take a few days during which we stick to a very specific protocol. This can have the benefit of squelching serious cravings for energy-killing sugar, salt, and fat—helping us to make the changes in our diets that we want permanent. But for now, let's turn to the secrets to nourishing and nurturing a happy body.

MAKING A HAPPY BELLY

Is your belly talking back to you? Does it call out to you in the most awkward moments? Have you been exercising and eating right but your belly hasn't changed shape—or worse it's expanded? Any and all of these are signs that you've got an unhappy belly. And it's time to take matters into your own hands . . . well, almost. It's important that if you have chronic (that means regularly occurring) digestive complaints that you speak to your doctor so that he or she can evaluate you to rule out anything being wrong, functionally speaking. If you are like so many of our clients, you will get the A-OK from your doctor, which can be bittersweet because it's great knowing there is nothing seriously wrong but you also know that your belly's blabbering is seriously causing disturbance in your life (and clothes!). And even if your doctor discovers something and prescribes a treatment protocol, eating right will be a core part of your plan.

Digestive complaints—gas, bloating, reflux, constipation, heartburn, irritable bowel, pain, diarrhea, or a wonderful combination of all or any of these—are signs of imbalances that your body wants you to tune in and correct, like yesterday. Your belly doesn't want to be sluggish, overworked and underpaid, or moving so fast it's out of control and leaves you spinning. Digestive disturbance means that nutrients aren't getting where they should—either to your cells for energy and repair work, or out of the body because they don't belong. So an unhappy belly is something that deserves your attention ASAP.

Don't be ashamed, for you're not alone. More than 80 million people in the United States suffer from digestive disorders, which happens to be the second leading cause of missed work behind the common cold. The role of digestion on energy levels is sorely overlooked, yet it literally could be "the guts" of moms' problems with low energy. An occasional bout of heartburn or constipation is often easy to tolerate and disregard, but these ailments are far too common these days and are doing more energy-depleting damage than we think. It doesn't matter what you take in (how good it is), if your inner machine isn't working, you won't achieve optimal energy. A healthy gut allows energy to flow. It acts as a center of gravity for all things energy related. In fact, your digestive system is way more than a processing plant for food; you'll soon come to learn that it's really the heart and soul of your immune system. It's pretty much the defender of your entire well-being.

First and foremost, digestion is your body's energy packer. It must work for the body to work. The best efforts fail in a compromised digestive system. We increasingly work with clients who forget to consider the health of their digestive system in addition to what they eat and how often they engage in physical activity. It may seem like common sense, but far too often the gut's overall health goes unnoticed until you've got a serious problem on your hands that makes it obvious, such as illness or disease. Although we have many barometers that we can use to tell us when something is wrong, such as blood pressure or heart rate, tummy trouble is a quick and easy telltale sign of the body experiencing an imbalance.

It's the body's way of saying, "Pay attention to what's bugging you!" Many of us can go long without figuring out the culprit to digestive problems, especially if those problems are covered up with frequent use of medications that dull symptoms, but do nothing to address the underlying culprit. What doesn't take long, however, is realizing how the unhappy belly makes us unhappy.

So it's really no surprise that the solution to our energy problems are sometimes as easy as fixing a poorly functioning gut. After all, your gut is arguably the most important ingredient in your overall energy equation. Your gut is also intimately involved in some intensely emotional business that factors into your energy equation: we rely upon our gut instinct to tell us the right thing to do! Who hasn't experienced a gut reaction to people who offend or delight us? Who hasn't felt sick before giving a speech or confronting a superior? We do a gut check when facing a challenge and congratulate ourselves when we display the intestinal fortitude, or guts, to take it on.

This is all for good reason, as your gut is synced up with your brain. Just think about how a bout of intense fear or panic can liquefy your innards—or, more commonly, when a cramp or brief wave of nausea alerts you to a nagging anxiety your mind had been working so hard to suppress. There's a good reason your gut and your brain communicate so seamlessly: every class of neurochemical produced in the first brain is also produced in the second.

Stress hormones present another kind of chemical that acts as the primary go-between for these two brains. When the brain detects any kind of threat—whether an impending layoff or a dustup with your spouse—it shoots stress hormones to your gut. Sensory nerves there respond by adjusting acid secretion and shutting down both appetite and digestion—a throwback to more dangerous times in our past, when we needed to summon all our resources to stand and fight, or flee. The result may be a nagging stomachache or a full-blown bout of gastrointestinal (GI) distress.

Suffice it to say our guts are very complex systems, which play into so much about us and our capacity to feel energetic.

The strategies presented in this chapter help rebuild a sick or malfunctioning digestive system, plus we'll give tips for those with added challenges such as lactose intolerance, acid-reflux, irritable bowel, gluten sensitivity, food allergies, and even migraines. Energy is often a casualty to other underlying conditions as well, such as anemia, thyroid issues, depression, sleep apnea, autoimmune disease, allergies, and diabetes.

Brief disclaimer: We're not here to help you formally diagnose any of these conditions if you do, in fact, suffer from one or more of them. We're here to equip you with the information you need so you can have that conversation with your doctor if you suspect that something else is going on to steal your energy. If you cannot get your energy level up after following the strategies in this book, we encourage you to seek medical help in targeting the problem. All too often hidden medical conditions can be overlooked, yet may have easy and quick remedies under a doctor's care. These strategies can be used in combination with therapies to treat an underlying condition.

Profile Alert! Anyone who identified themselves as Profile 1 (The Medicine Cabinet), should digest every sentence of this chapter. We also think that Profile 2 (The Mom Zombie) and Profile 5 (The Dead Battery) would do well to read through this chapter slowly. Think about your habits, behaviors, and personal conditions that could be the main instigators of your energy woes.

The Guts of the Matter

In the hectic pace of everyday life, the health—and the mechanics—of your digestive system is not on your mind. But it's undoubtedly something that none of us can afford to ignore. Once you've taken your last bite of a meal, you probably don't think about what's going on inside from your brain all the way down to your bowels.

You may have drawn the curtain on your eating for the moment, but the show has just begun for your gut, and it will take between nine hours and a day or two for the food you just ate to be fully digested. During that time, your stomach and small intestine break your food down into molecules that the small intestine's thin lining can absorb, allowing essential nutrients—the energy stream that fuels every cell in your body—to enter your bloodstream. The lower part of your small intestine then wrings out the water remaining in your meal and ushers it into your colon, which funnels it into your bloodstream to help keep you hydrated.

As straightforward as this process sounds, the seemingly simple chore of digestion depends on a finely orchestrated series of muscular contractions, chemical secretions, and electrical signals all along the 30-foot-long gastrointestinal tract. And there's plenty you can do to keep this operation running smoothly.

Digestive health is the center of gravity for all other points of health in the body. When out of balance, sick, or diseased, virtually every other system and organ gets negatively affected, triggering scores of problems you wouldn't normally or intuitively link directly to the digestive tract. As noted earlier, irritable bowel syndrome (IBS), for instance, is one of the most common intestinal disorders, affecting about 10 to 15 percent of people in North America alone. Up to 20 percent of people have symptoms of IBS, such as abdominal pain and altered bowel habits, although less than half of them see a doctor for their symptoms—most of which interfere with normal life and feelings of energy. But what few people talk about is that getting a diagnosis of IBS requires so much energy investment. First, you see your doctor, who then usually wants to run a few tests and he or she may ask you to keep a food journal. You may have to see a specialist if tests don't turn up anything, which then eventually leads to the following: "The good news is there is nothing wrong with you (functionally), so it must be irritable bowel syndrome." And then you will be told to work on stress, diet, lifestyle, and perhaps you'll be given some symptom-relieving recommendations to try, such as fiber, medication for acid reflux, and so on.

A Fine Balance

Generally speaking, we perform two broad physiological functions in charging and running our battery. First, we take in and absorb nutrients, and second we expel waste products of that energy metabolism. It's the yin and yang of energy metabolism, similar to what we do when we cook in the kitchen: first we make a great meal but then we have to clean up. We excrete our body's waste products (clean up our kitchens) mostly when we visit the bathroom, but also to a lesser degree when we breathe, sweat, cut our hair, and trim our nails. Everyday physiological processes such as energy production, digestion, and hormone synthesis create waste products that, if not discarded, interfere with the function of our internal organs.

Most of these wastes are the by-products of the air we breathe and the food we eat. However, our intestinal tracts are full of bacteria and yeast that also produce waste. These bacteria and yeast are often called gut flora or intestinal microbes. Some of these bacteria are highly beneficial. They assist in the digestion of some vitamins and they play a significant role in our immune response. About 100 trillion (three pounds) of these bacteria live in the intestinal tracts of virtually every human on earth. In fact, we have more of these microbes living in our intestinal tract than we have cells in our body (only about 80 trillion). These bacteria are either good for you, bad for you, or neutral.

The good bacteria are often called probiotics (a term that means "for life") because of the role they play in keeping us healthy. These good bacteria produce substances such as acetic acid, which helps to destroy harmful bacteria. Two examples of these good bacteria are *Lactobacillus acidophilus* and *Bifidobacteria bifidum*. We also have bad intestinal flora. Some examples of bad flora are salmonella and *Candida albicans*, a yeast that can cause an infection when it grows out of control. This is the same yeast that causes some of us to get vaginal yeast infections. These bad flora are constantly taking in nutrients and creating wastes in the form of indol, skatol, and methane. Methane is an internally produced toxin that results in gas and bloating. Long-term production of these internal toxins can lead to a weakened immune system, inflammation, and a slower metabolic rate. Obviously, we want the good bacteria to be more prevalent than the bad bacteria. We can't ever eradicate all the bad bacteria—it's a part of life. But if the balance is upset, we see an increased risk for digestive problems, impaired immune system, skin problems (resulting from digestive disturbances—our skin is our other major excretory organ and remember stuff that's meant to get out of the body will find a way to get out!), and other potential health issues.

If you've ever had food poisoning, you know your gut is an uncompromising vigilante. When a nasty microbe hitchhikes a ride into the body on the back of real food, the gut quickly recognizes the interloper and strong-arms it to the nearest exit. To make the ID in the first place, it calls upon a reliable army of sentries, millions of immune system cells residing in its walls.

If the fact that the gut plays a major role in immunity sounds surprising, consider that the whole purpose of the immune system is to differentiate what's you from what's not you. Then consider that every day, you introduce pounds of foreign material—your daily bread—into your gut. The immune system has to decide what's okay to let through and what's not, so it makes sense to headquarter that process right where the food comes in.

This powerful system gears up from day one. A newborn's gastrointestinal tract is entirely germ free, but immediately after birth, pioneering bacteria begin to colonize it. The first few years of life, everyone's gut develops a unique extended family of bacterial species, determined in part by genetics and in part by diet, hygiene, medication use, and the bacteria colonizing those around us. Perhaps bacteria's most important job: stimulating and training the body's immune system and, by its overwhelming presence, crowding out more harmful critters.

The specific microbial mix (your gut contains thousands of species of bacteria) you wind up with has a big impact on your health. Besides making you more resistant to disease, the balance (or lack thereof) of microbes in your gut may lower your risk of obesity or influence your risk of autoimmune disorders such as rheumatoid arthritis, multiple sclerosis, psoriasis, and inflammatory bowel disease. Clearly, this extended family deserves coddling.

Probiotics: Hype or Help?

It's hard to imagine that we each host billions of live bacteria in our digestive tract that colonize by replicating quickly and massively, but it's true. What's even more fascinating is that different bacteria live in different places based on what they desire as a home environment. Think of a native Montanan versus a New York City resident—some like crowds and feed off the energy of the crowd, the noise doesn't bother them, the pollution isn't a major deterrent, and they've adapted to the types of food available, whereas others need wide open space. They preferentially choose pure air and hunting for their food, and they are okay if they only see a crowd on holidays or if they happen to travel. By the same token, a person who lives in Montana will have a different gut flora than someone who lives in New York—or Tokyo—for that matter.

There are many more bacteria in the large intestine versus the small intestine (100,000:1), as it is significantly less acidic; another way of saying this is to remember that your lower GI prefers to be more alkaline. The small intestine contains more digestive enzymes, has more movement (peristalsis), and generates more antimicrobial chemicals (for example probiotics acting on fiber can create an acidic by-product that functions like an antibiotic). Thus, because bacteria have different preferences, what we eat and as a result the environment in each area of our digestive tract will either encourage or discourage the bacteria to inhabit and flourish in their respective geography.

Outside factors, in addition to what we eat, affect bacteria balance ("gut flora"). Antibiotics ("anti" meaning against, and "biotic" meaning bacteria vs. "pro" meaning for, or good) get rid of the good with the bad so even one dose of antibiotics can upset the desirable ratio of bacteria. This doesn't happen immediately, but it does occur exponentially week after week due to how quickly bacteria replicate. So if we don't replenish the good bacteria, the bad can get an advantage right off the bat once the antibiotic's action wears off. Many of us were given antibiotics frequently as children (to treat ear and throat infections) or as young adults for skin problems. It's very common for doctors today to treat adult patients complaining of GI problems and learn that their issues stem from a lifetime of periodic or even chronic antibiotic use that caused an imbalance in their gut flora. This isn't as uncommon as you might think. By the time an individual reaches her late 20s, she can experience digestive problems that are then exacerbated by the inclusion of birth control pills and/or poor dietary choices over the previous decade. What's more, today's food and water technology makes it difficult to avoid getting secondhand exposure to antibiotics by eating animals and even drinking water in some places that have been treated with antibiotics.

As an aside, one key side effect of bacteria imbalance is a tendency to bloat around the middle and gain abdominal weight despite good dietary and activity practices. Additionally, we continue to be intrigued by research exploring the link between bacteria imbalance and obesity, for there is some compelling evidence that deserves further exploration. Imagine being able to control or treat obesity by simply changing the balance of intestinal bacteria, or even the types of bacteria present. Future research will bear this out.

So how do we get the balance back? Probiotics are found in food and in supplement form. Let's discuss the foods first. Before probiotics became the food trend they are today, reliable food sources of probiotics included fermented foods such as kimchi, raw sauerkraut, pickles, miso/natto, cultured vegetables, yogurts, aged cheese, and kefirs. Today, a rapidly growing number of food products (not fermented foods) are marketing themselves as containing probiotics. This raises two issues: (1) can/do they support live bacteria in their product (a lot of them note the amount of live bacteria at the time of manufacture—not at the time of consumption), and (2) do they contain a strain that has proven to be effective? Although we don't need to be eating foods that added probiotics to them—there is no danger, and in fact they could do good if the probiotic is viable (live)—but the question is about need and dietary diversity. We don't need cereals that contain probiotics—our cereals can be our fiber and other nutrient sources and if we want probiotics we can eat some yogurt with the cereal. We can choose from the aforementioned list of foods that naturally contain probiotics. If we are allergic to one and don't like the taste of another, we can move on to a different one on the list.

Some companies are making different versions of foods that naturally contain probiotics. Many of these are worth exploring, especially if dietary preferences or intolerances restrict certain foods (such as dairy). But also be a knowledgeable consumer and be wary of marketing or food trends. For example, of the numerous yogurts being marketed for their probiotics, many contain higher than necessary (and higher than healthy) amounts of added sugar in the name of getting in probiotics. Yogurt comes from milk so it will naturally have milk sugar, but it doesn't need added sugar. Find out how many probiotics are in these specially created probiotic yogurts (many don't say on the label) as opposed to a regular yogurt as opposed to a frozen yogurt marketed for its probiotic content. Per serving, most of them are similar, so make your choice based on what your palate desires and skip the sugar-coated probiotic unless you were going for something sugar-coated anyway! And if you don't want to do all this work—you can refer to the AKA list of approved products at www.AshleyKoffRD.com.

For individuals without the health issues described above and who have never take antibiotics, routine probiotic consumption through food should be sufficient to maintain bacteria balance. However, for those seeking to address health issues impacted by bacteria imbalance, a probiotic supplement will likely have the best therapeutic benefit in addition to dietary modifications. Supplements can guarantee that one gets a probiotic dosage sufficient to address symptoms. The necessary quantity ranges with the type and severity of the health issue.

A word on probiotics in supplement form: they are not all created equal. The type of probiotic, "strain specificity," is critical when it comes to the selection of a probiotic supplement to address a health issue. Clinical research, as well as anecdotal reports from practitioners, helps to validate which strains demonstrate greater effectiveness than others. For example, *B. infantis* is one of a few strains found to improve all symptoms of irritable bowel syndrome. Some strains of *L. bulgaricus* have been shown to aid in lowering cholesterol.

Additionally, supplements, lacking government oversight of probiotic production may not contain what they say they do. Also, the bacteria may not be alive at the time you take the supplement despite it being packaged alive (probiotics are very heat sensitive which is why most require refrigeration). In 2005, *Consumer Reports* found 40 percent of the probiotics tested contained significantly fewer live microbes than the label promised. So caution with product selection is recommended. For a list of brand recommendations, visit www.AshleyKoffRD.com and check out *The Probiotics Revolution* by Gary Huffnagle.

And just because we put the good guys in there, doesn't mean they have what it takes to do battle successfully. What tools do they need? How can we cultivate a friendly environment for good bacteria? More and more we're hearing about prebiotics, which are defined as non-digestible food ingredients that stimulate the growth and/or activity of healthy bacteria in the digestive system. It helps to think of prebiotics as precursors to healthy bacteria—they provide raw materials that the good bacteria prefer to have available in order to thrive. Typically, prebiotics are carbohydrates but they may include noncarbohydrates. The most prevalent forms of prebiotics are nutritionally classed as soluble fiber. Many forms of dietary fiber exhibit some level of prebiotic effect. Examples of foods containing prebiotics include raw chicory root, raw Jerusalem artichoke, raw garlic, raw leeks, raw onions, raw asparagus, raw wheat bran, cooked whole-wheat flour, and raw banana. In addition to including prebiotic fibers in the diet, we can also create a more hospitable environment by focusing on choosing foods and beverages that help promote a more alkaline environment in the intestines (See Chapter 5).

Bottom line: while just adding probiotics may not be the magic bullet or cure-all, they are definitely part of the solution!

Original Sources of Pro- and Prebiotics:

- Probiotics: kimchi, raw sauerkraut, yogurt, dairy kefir, coconut water kefir, fermented soy (tempeh, miso, natto)

- Prebiotics: Jerusalem artichoke (sunchokes), chicory root, asparagus, oats, raw honey, barley, flaxseeds (ground), onions

---

Common Conditions That Cramp Your Digestive Style

No one gets to 100 percent perfection in anything. Repeat: no one gets 100 percent perfection. This is especially true in the digestive-wellness department. So aim high but not for perfection (let's say 80 to 90 percent most of the time). Digestive wellness isn't something you achieve and then can forget about, quickly reverting back to your old habits. People will say, "So I've been avoiding refined flour products and coffee for three months and feel great; can I have it again, now?" The answer is maybe yes, and you can choose to test the waters to see if you can go back to having something you gave up. However, keep a few things in mind. For most of us, digestive problems didn't develop in just three months—likely they were years in the making (remember your college eating/drinking plan, or after-school outings in junior high?). And while giving something up for forever seems dramatic, equally dramatic is the idea that having something means that you have it every day. When we remove different items as part of therapeutic treatment we are doing so for two reasons: to reduce known irritants and to identify potential intolerances. The latter may never come back into your eating regimen but the former may make their way back—infrequently—once your system is no longer in its irritated state. That said, let's go back to the initial sentence: " . . . and feel great." Why is it that if you feel great, now is the time when you want to make changes or revert back? How great does great feel? Perhaps you don't even need to try an old food source. Maybe it's about trying something new. Instead of the coffee, maybe you try coconut water or herbal tea. Or instead of pasta you try quinoa, kamut, or millet—if these were good enough to make strong bodies of the Greeks, Chinese, and Aztecs, perhaps they will do the same for you, too.

Following is a quick rundown of common conditions that are linked to digestive issues. Use this as a guide to understanding the basics to these energy-killing culprits and discuss your unique concerns and questions with your doctor.

Autoimmune Diseases (e.g., rheumatoid arthritis, fibromyalgia, lupus, multiple sclerosis): Although these are not technically "digestive disorders" we must mention them because not only are they prevalent among millions of women today, but they are conditions that can indeed cramp a digestive style. Anyone who suffers from an autoimmune disorder has a system that, for whatever reason, is attacking itself. Such a hostile environment does not bode well for the digestive tract that aims to achieve nutrient and energy balance. It's common for people with an autoimmune disease to simultaneously suffer from food intolerances and digestive disorders that require unique attention to diet.

Celiac Disease: This condition entails an allergic reaction within the inner lining of the small intestine to proteins (gluten) that are present in wheat, rye, barley, and, to a lesser extent, oats due to cross-contamination in production. The body's immune response causes inflammation that destroys the lining of the small intestine, which then reduces the absorption of dietary nutrients and can lead to symptoms and signs of nutritional, vitamin, and mineral deficiencies.

Some people may not have celiac disease but are still sensitive to gluten. For both the gluten-sensitive or, at the extreme, intolerant person, following a gluten-free nutrition plan is about a lot more than just removing gluten from the diet. To heal the digestive system (and maintain a healthy digestive system), as well as to reduce the risk of other chronic diseases and to maintain a healthy weight, it is critical to consider all aspects of the diet. This means paying attention to quality, quantity, nutrient balance, and frequency—all of which were discussed in Chapter 5. Unfortunately, the surge in "G-free" products has resulted in a glut of options that wouldn't rank high on the nutrient meter and could just trigger other energy imbalances. It's shocking how many G-free products, for instance, contain chemicals, artificial ingredients, and excessive amounts of sugar and unhealthy fats—as if gluten-free automatically means healthy or healthiest. What's more, some of these ingredients can be irritating, so you eliminate one problem (gluten) but haven't addressed the overall health/energy issue fully. For everyone, especially someone who suffers from allergies, autoimmune disease, or other indications that the body is challenged, we need quality food choices—period! Anyone choosing to or having to follow a gluten-free diet should aim to make organic and whole-food choices as often as possible.

Chronic constipation or diarrhea: Both of these ailments are very common yet there are numerous possible reasons causing either one, including IBS, medications, infections, etc. The common denominator here is an imbalance in the body's movement of food through the digestive tract. Somewhere, there's an imbalance and the result is constipation or diarrhea—and in some cases, an alternating of the two. Many moms don't even acknowledge a change in their bowels until they begin to discuss it with girlfriends or watch Dr. Oz.

Gastroesophageal Reflux Disease (GERD): GERD is a condition in which the liquid content of the stomach regurgitates (backs up, or refluxes) into the esophagus. Some people reflux up food or liquids, while others reflux acid, so in truth GERD does not always equal acid reflux. But stomach liquids usually contain stomach acid and the enzyme pepsin, both of which can inflame and damage the lining of the esophagus. The refluxed liquid also may contain bile that has backed up into the stomach from the duodenum, which is the first part of the small intestine that attaches to the stomach. The acid is believed to be the most injurious component of the refluxed liquid, though pepsin and bile also may cause damage. Lots of medications are available today to help combat GERD, both over-the-counter and by prescription.

But if we just turn to a drug, we may be missing something. The body's normal function is not to reflux (unless it is helping us in a moment of trauma to avoid choking or to get rid of something that it detects as bad for us). If you are having reflux routinely it means that the body is seriously trying to tell you something. It could be that you're producing too much stomach acid, but a lot of people actually have too little acid in the stomach. Too much food or eating too quickly? Food intolerances? Gravity working against you (lying down after eating)? As you can see, there are many things that could be factors, and medication addresses just one—reducing the acid. So if it isn't your specific problem or your entire problem, you may not get the full fix. Let's review some ideas to try before or in conjunction with a medication:

- Keep the digestive tract *under*whelmed: eat small, frequent (about every three hours) meals and chew your food well. Let your mouth do some of the work so your esophagus and stomach get what they need, how they need it!

- Incorporate plant-based digestive enzyme supplements with your meals, especially when you eat animal proteins. Plant enzymes can help break down the food.

- Already have esophageal irritation? Add an L-glutamine supplement: this amino acid may aid tissue recovery.

- Get plenty of probiotics naturally from foods (e.g., yogurt with *Lactobacillus* and *Bifidobacterium*) and/or take a high-quality supplement containing live cultures (e.g., Align with Bifantis).

- Shoot for more omega-3s, naturally found in wild cold-water fish or taken as a supplement. Omega-3s may help reduce any inappropriate inflammation of the digestive tract.

- Chew deglycyrrhizinated licorice between meals (we know, it's a mouthful of a word, but it is commonly referred to by the acronym DGL). This can work as an acid-reflux aid. Try mastic gum, which has antibacterial properties.

- Try taking magnesium citrate or glycinate before bed to improve the movement of food and waste through your digestive tract.

- Avoid lying down or going to bed right after eating or drinking. Give yourself a two-to-three-hour window ideally to allow for digestion of food to get it past the stomach.

Insulin insensitivity and resistance: Millions of Americans are increasingly getting diagnosed as insulin insensitive or resistant, a prelude to diabetes as well as a key sign that the body's energy equations are out of balance. Here's the short story on how it happens: If you overconsume refined or poor quality carbs, your glucose level will rise sharply, but soon fall back quickly. (Note: Other issues could also be at play, such as deficiencies of necessary nutrients; not enough chromium, for example, can inhibit insulin absorption.) When this happens, you experience a true energy low. At the same time, you usually experience a craving for more carbohydrates to bring your blood sugar back up, which will offset the general feeling of malaise characterized by shakiness, fatigue, brain fog, and dizziness that go with low blood sugar or hypoglycemia. Habitual energy imbalances like this set off a repetitive pattern of quick rises and drops in blood sugar levels, which can challenge your pancreas and liver. Both of these organs manage insulin—your body's chief energy hormone, which gets released from the pancreas upon eating and escorts glucose out of the blood and into the tissues. As you can imagine, when this pattern repeats itself over time, your whole body's energy metabolism can begin to falter, and soon enough you might find yourself in a prediabetic state on the road to diabetes. The good news about gaining control over this chaos is that it can be as simple as gaining control of your diet and related lifestyle risk factors like excess weight and smoking.

Intolerances: Anyone who has the unfortunate experience of consuming a problematic food knows that it's an energy killer. Food allergies, for instance, are on the rise today, especially among children. The number of kids with food allergies went up 18 percent from 1997 to 2007, according to the U.S. Centers for Disease Control and Prevention. This term can be misconstrued, however. A true food allergy is an abnormal response to food that is triggered by a specific reaction of the immune system and expressed by certain, often characteristic, symptoms. Other kinds of reactions to foods that are not food allergies include food intolerances (such as lactose intolerance), food poisoning, and toxic reactions. Food intolerance is also an abnormal response to food, and its symptoms can resemble those of food allergy. Food intolerance, however, is far more prevalent, occurs in a variety of diseases, and is triggered by several different mechanisms that are distinct from the immunological reaction responsible for food allergy. The most important thing to keep in mind is that the body, when irritated, will appear intolerant to most of that which is presented because it is trying to get our attention. It's irritated to the point that anything that goes in will be seen as an annoyance. So working on digestive wellness overall as opposed to troubleshooting certain intolerances is the prescription. In other words, if you are lactose intolerant and also have other intolerances, just switching to lactose-free products won't necessarily heal your system.

Irritable Bowel Syndrome (IBS): As already noted, IBS is one of the most common ailments of the bowel (intestines). What can be frustrating about IBS is that it's not linked to any structural defects. In other words, it's a functional disorder. If you are personally familiar with IBS, then you know very well how much it can hamper quality of life. Many studies have concluded that the constant intake of food additives and the ingestion of pesticides, chemicals, and dyes can cause irritation to the intestinal tract and/or an imbalance of the intestinal bacteria, resulting in inflammation or symptoms of IBS.

Lactose Intolerance: If you can't digest and absorb the sugar in milk (lactose), you're said to be "lactose intolerant." It makes eating dairy products all the more challenging and painful. Your GI will scream "oh no!" and you'll feel it with gas, bloating, urgent/uncontrolled bowel movements, and general discomfort. The first cure for lactose intolerance is to simply avoid the foods that trigger the problem (ahem, anything containing milk). Depending on the severity of your intolerance, you may be able to consume hard cheeses, fermented dairy, and sheep or goat's milk products versus cow's milk. That said, whenever consuming dairy you want to consume the highest quality. Just because lactose-free products are available, if they have a lot of sugar or artificial ingredients, they may help you with the lactose issue but be poor for overall energy and health. Lactose-free products are widely available today, as are supplements to further help you digest milk-containing foods and beverages. Lots of people don't realize they are lactose intolerant until they no longer want to tolerate its awful side effects and are ready to get to the bottom of their discomfort by zeroing in on the culprit. Half the battle is just coming to terms with being lactose intolerant, and then doing what you can to minimize your exposure to lactose.

Small Intestinal Bacterial Overgrowth (SIBO): SIBO refers to a condition in which abnormally large numbers of bacteria are present in the small intestine and the types of bacteria resemble the kind typically found only in the colon (large intestine). This encroachment of bacteria can cause gas, bloating, cramps, diarrhea, and constipation. SIBO may also contribute to food allergies and nutritional deficiencies. The good news is that it's easy to test for and responds well to proper treatment.

Secrets to a Happy Belly

In addition to any specific prescriptions that a doctor would advise that you follow to heal a sick digestive system, be it a diagnosed problem such as IBS or just chronic constipation with no definitive culprit, all of the following suggestions will help you to maintain as healthy a gut as possible. Also keep in mind that the other things we outline in this book—eating quality food in good proportions, limiting alcohol consumption, getting a good night's sleep, and incorporating regular exercise into your routine—are important to maintaining your happy belly.

Remember: your ultimate goal in soothing a troubled tummy is to get clearer intuitive signals. When something really bugs you, your second brain will let you know loud and clear. Use the following strategies in combination with any of the ones described above to match your unique issues. And again, discuss any protocol with your physician.

Think slow and steady: A rushed meal is out of sync with the creeping pace of the gut. In the last chapter you learned why eating every three hours is good for your energy metabolism, and good for your gut. This approach also helps you to avoid overeating, as your next meal won't be too far away. Our bodies prepare to eat at the mere thought, sight, and smell of good food. The digestive process actually starts before we take our first bite, as our brains send signals to our stomachs and salivary glands to secrete chemicals that will help break down food. Chew your food well so your gut doesn't have to work as hard to break it down. Eat slowly to avoid gulping air, which will make you gassy, bloated and—thanks to the mind's payback to the body—irritable.

Mind your manners: Chewing gum, smoking, drinking through a straw, and talking while you're eating can all cause you to swallow excess air, leaving you bloated and uncomfortable.

Find your inner balance: Gut-friendly bacteria use fiber as their main food source, hence the recommendation to eat plenty of fruits, vegetables, and whole grains, such as oats, barley, whole wheat, and popcorn. Fiber also aids the passage of food and waste through the gut. Aim for over 20 grams of fiber a day. But again, go slowly: increasing your fiber intake too quickly can cause gas and bloating.

In the next chapter, we'll offer some ideas on how to do a detox correctly—one that supports your digestive health rather than hinders it. Many of today's detox diets, or colonic cleaners, will wipe out the good bacteria and cause an overgrowth of the bad bacteria.

Don't be too sweet: Keep this in mind the next time you go for a treat. Sugars, dried fruit, sweeteners, and juice are treats that are not friendly for many digestive systems. Carbonated drinks on top of excess sugar such as sodas can make your stomach puffy, bloated, and distended. Keep it simple—stick to water with lemon, added organic frozen fruit, and herbal teas.

Follow the rules of the restroom: Unfortunately, toilet seats recline us back because they are too high for most of us. Solution: lean forward and rest your chest on your lap as if you're trying to read a newspaper on the floor (you can also place something to read on the floor if that helps). This avoids pushing or straining to have a bowel movement, and puts your body into a more squatlike position. In a squatting position, the abdominal wall and the bowels are fully supported for more complete elimination.

Turn a digestive frown upside down: Having a bad belly day? Cooked fruits and vegetables, such as a baked apple, steamed spinach, etc., may work better than raw. Avoid known gastric irritants. Lower your intake of animal fats (dairy, beef, etc.) and replace it with plant fats such as hemp seeds, hemp oil, chia, or flaxseed oil. Eat smaller portions, and try digestive enzymes. Also some people do better with purees and liquids on these days—just make sure you still make nutrient-dense and nutrient-balanced choices.

Spice things up: Spices don't just make your food taste good, they're important for your overall health, too. Ginger and turmeric have anti-inflammatory properties, while caraway, cumin, and cinnamon play a role in digestion and can help with weight management. Adding different spices to your meals and snacks can help spice things up . . . the right way.

Respect what your gut has to say: Even the most finely tuned machine has its quirks—if certain foods trigger GI problems for you, avoid them. Common heartburn culprits: acidic, spicy, and fatty foods; caffeinated and carbonated drinks; chocolate; and onions. Make it a goal to replace known gastric irritants with gastric healers, so you're not just getting rid of irritants.

Notorious gas producers include beans, onions, and cruciferous vegetables such as cauliflower, cabbage, and radishes. (These veggies are loaded with vital nutrients, so don't shun them altogether, but enjoy them in small doses.) The same goes for packaged low-carb treats and other foods containing artificial sweeteners—especially the sweetener sorbitol.

Bust the bloat: A probiotic can help you get rid of stomach bloating and make your middle area look smaller. It also will help the body process carbs and support the immune system.

Breathe into your belly: Meditation, yoga, deep breathing, and other practices that encourage mindful relaxation encourage the body to be less sensitive to stress. Plus these practices force more oxygen into your body, which will amp up your energy metabolism and streamline your systems. Deep breathing, using the muscles of your diaphragm (you should feel your belly expand and deflate with each inhale and exhale), can also help calm your mind and release tension in your abdominal muscles, easing indigestion. It will also further help flush toxins and inflammatory molecules from your body. Another way to calm the body's autonomic nervous system—which regulates digestion, among other things—is through progressive muscle relaxation, tightening and then relaxing small groups of muscles beginning in your toes and working your way up to your face. (More ideas on this will be presented in Part IV.)

Balance your pH: An overly acidic system can wreak havoc not just on your digestive system but also your bones and skin. How so? Bad bacteria and viruses thrive in an acidic environment, and in order for the body to maintain its preferred pH of about 7.4, it will remove calcium from the bone to alkalinize itself. So while our body needs acid in the stomach, the rest of the digestive tract and resulting urine is meant to be alkaline for optimal health.

Things that contribute to excess acidity:

- Excess animal protein: if you eat animal protein, exercise portion control and make sure to balance the protein with plenty of alkaline food choices (see page 152).

- Chronic stress, lack of sleep, dehydration, unresolved anger, overall depletion: tough times happen, but learning to relax and replenish the system is critical.

- Artificial additives: sweeteners and preservatives can add extra hydrogen or acidic ions to the system, producing inappropriate acidity in the body.

- Unnaturally white foods: white sugar and white flour are acid forming.

You can help alkalinize your system by reducing the acidifiers and increasing your alkalinizers. Here are some ideas:

- Add lemon to your water: a weak acid, lemon can actually alkalinize.

- Go green: include more vegetables in your diet, such as parsley, seaweeds, kale, celery, and spinach.

- Choose whole and sprouted grains (even more alkaline forming): standouts include quinoa, millet, and amaranth.

- Play around with incorporating these potent alkalinizers: sesame seeds (great source of calcium), fresh coconut, almonds, apple-cider vinegar, sea salt, cayenne, and watermelon.

Go Pro, and Avoid the Anti: Look for yogurts and plain kefir, as well as other fermented foods that contain strains of *Lactobacillus* and *Bifidobacteria*. In addition to protecting against colds and flu and promoting healthful bacteria, probiotics can help relieve diarrhea caused by infection or antibiotics, irritable bowel syndrome, or Crohn's disease. Watch out for antibiotics. Though you may need these on occasion to treat an infection, overusing antibiotics can disrupt your gut's microflora. They kill not only the pathogens causing your ailment but also good bacteria.

Avoid inflammatory foods: While avoiding inflammatory foods is always a good idea, it's especially important if you're trying to heal an unhappy belly. Use the table on the next page as a quick guide to what you should buy. Eating in this manner will reduce inflammation and help your belly get back to normal.

Consume as often as possible:	Avoid as much as possible:
Foods that can be found in nature	Food products (no trans fats, partially hydrogenated oils, high-fructose corn syrup, dyes)
Foods with recognizable ingredients	Foods with ingredients you cannot define
Whole, high-quality foods	Completely ready-to-eat meals from poor-quality ingredients, preservatives
New foods daily and on a seasonal basis	Same thing every day
Whole fruits and vegetables—skin, pulp, and cells are packed with nutrients	Fruit products, including juices
Vegetable sources of protein—good sources of fiber and valuable nutrients	Animal proteins exclusively as a way to avoid carbs (quality carbs are an essential part of any healthy nutritional plan)
Vegetables at meals and snacks to satisfy hunger	More animal protein or fat to feel full

Meals full of natural colors	One color or colorless meals
Fruits and vegetables with dark-colored flesh or leaves	Vegetables without color (e.g., iceberg lettuce, white potatoes)
Fresh and frozen organic fruits and vegetables	Canned, dried, and processed conventional fruits and vegetables
A variety of whole grains	Refined grains (flours, white bread, crackers, etc.) or flour-based carbohydrates at every meal
Wheat-free grains such as quinoa, amaranth, teff, buckwheat, oats, rice, and wild rice	Wheat every time you want a grain
Organic, locally grown, hormone-free, preservative-free foods	Chemicals
Water, herbal teas, healing tonics	Nutrient-poor, high-calorie, or artificially sweetened beverages
Dishes that are inherently flavorful by cooking with spices and herbs	Foods hidden beneath sauces of unknown origin

ADDITIONAL HEALTH CONSIDERATIONS

Just about any medical condition can cause a major disruption in your energy metabolism, but for us to address each one individually would take up an entire library of books. However, we didn't want to ignore that medical conditions—and what you're doing to treat them—can seriously affect your energy. Below is a snapshot of some strategies to consider if the advice in this book doesn't enhance your energy or if you know you are dealing with a larger medical condition.

Mind the medications: Virtually all medications, whether they are over-the-counter or prescribed, can change your body's natural energy metabolism. Common energy-depleting culprits include proton pump inhibitors (e.g., Prilosec, Nexium, Prevacid, etc.), birth control, antibiotics, sleep medications such as Ambien, SSRIs for depression (e.g., Prozac, Zoloft, Paxil, etc.), allergy medications, pain relievers, and drugs to boost bone density. Even cosmetic injections and treatments for skin conditions such as acne and psoriasis can be energy depleting. Be sure to discuss your concerns about medication affecting your energy levels with your physician. It's possible that another medication can be prescribed that won't affect your energy as much.

Heed hormonal hang-ups: The get-help message applies here, too. We'll explore how stress does a number on our hormones in Chapter 10, but take note: if you cannot regulate your hormones—from digestive ones to those that control your mood, menstruation, metabolism, and even your perceived level of stress—then you cannot regulate your energy. As women, we worry so much about the illnesses related to hormonal imbalances rather than considering what could be *influencing* the hormones to begin with. Remember, hormones are our body's main couriers. They send messages back and forth, so everything about energy is wrapped around hormones. Like pain, when hormones are off, it's relatively easy to go into a "crazy mode" (i.e., *I feel like I'm having an* *out-of-body experience!*); or a sad and frustrated mode (i.e., *I feel like I am doing everything right but not getting results!*). Either mode can make us susceptible to grabbing at proverbial straws—emptying our wallets in front of infomercials, trying new plans touted in magazines or among friends, and so on. Having an open conversation about your hormones with your doctor is critical, and you need to keep these conversations going. All of the strategies in this book will help you to optimize your body's main hormonal cycles. Some cycles may require calling in heavier artillery in the form of hormone-replacement therapy, which is a decision you have to make with your doctor's help. Just as there can be no rhyme or reason to experiencing hormonal hang-ups, there's really no definitive cure for hormonal challenges. It must entail a combination of therapies that include diet, exercise, and sometimes supplements and medication. (For more, see Kathy's Energy Advice on page 157.)

Test your thyroid: Your thyroid is your master metabolism hormone. If it's out of balance, guess what: so are you. Your metabolism will be running amok and taking your energy with it. An underperforming thyroid (hypothyroidism) is one of the most underdiagnosed conditions in America, yet it's incredibly common—especially among women. Common symptoms include depression, muscle cramps, joint pain, dry skin, thinning hair, low sex drive, menstrual problems, weight gain or difficulty losing weight, constipation, a "foggy" mind, and of course fatigue. Although all of these symptoms may be blamed on the aging process itself, a low-functioning thyroid can also be at play. It's believed that 20 percent of all women have a lazy thyroid, but only half of women get diagnosed. More bad news: there is no single symptom or test that can properly diagnose hypothyroidism. To arrive at a trustworthy diagnosis, you'll need to look at your symptoms in addition to blood tests. And to fix a thyroid problem you'll also need to look at the whole picture. This means making sure you get key nutrients needed for your thyroid to function, including vitamins and minerals such as selenium, iodine, zinc, vitamins A and D, and the omega-3 fats. It also means supporting your adrenal glands by reducing your stress load. And it may mean going on some type of thyroid hormone-replacement therapy. Your doctor will be able to tailor a protocol specific to you.

Don't dodge a diagnosis: If you have any inkling that something else is going on with your body beyond a condition remedied through traditional diet and lifestyle choices, speak up!

Plan a visit with your doctor and have that conversation. If you don't know what you're dealing with, you can't begin to take proper action. Energy woes can be blamed on conditions as straightforward as anemia (low red blood cells that provide much-needed, energy-infusing oxygen) to those as complex as fibromyalgia, rheumatoid arthritis, or menopause. If you suffer from migraines, do what you can to manage them with attention to dietary triggers, sufficient sleep, and medication when necessary. If you're an insomniac (and Chapter 9 isn't enough to cure you), then ask your doctor about visiting a sleep lab. You may have sleep apnea, which can be easily treated and which will allow you to get your life—and energy—back! In sum: get help.

THE BOTTOM LINE: PHYSIOLOGY FIRST

It's pretty simple: if the body doesn't have what it needs to function, it won't do so or it won't do so optimally. Depending on your unique physiological needs and concerns, you may require a medication to treat an underlying condition. Or you may just need to overhaul your diet and exercise more. Either way, it's important to deal with your energy issues—large or small—as these indicate a problem with your overall health.

If you're experiencing the pain and discomfort of a chronic or acute condition, don't let it lead you astray in the energy-saving realm. When we are in pain, we may eat poorly and forgo exercise—the very ingredients needed for our bodies to heal. If it gets to this point, you should talk with your doctor about what options there are for you.

And if you do reach for help in the form of a medication it should only be temporary, as medication can perpetuate a cycle that promotes the pain and drains the energy. And bear in mind that when you do take medications, you are asking your body to rely on that medication rather than its own tools. Drugs can oftentimes stimulate other conditions. You don't want to trade one problem for another. If you take iron supplements to treat anemia, for example, the iron can trigger constipation and require another set of medications or nonpharmaceutical strategies to avoid the constipation.

A disease or symptom is a flashing sign that energy equations have been disrupted beneath. If we only give medications to make the body "correct" again, then we may miss looking at the core issue causing the problem. And we may miss the ultimate solution. For example, if you have diabetes, you can use insulin or sugar-free foods to correct your blood sugar, but what about eating better quality foods to begin with? What about getting key nutrients found in whole, natural foods?

Diabetes isn't just about too much sugar in the blood or about not enough insulin; these are symptomatic of the deeper problem of chronic inflammation, which is a risk factor for so many diseases. So if you reduce your sugar by exchanging sugary foods and beverages for sugar-free ones, but don't address the quality of your overall diet, you still have risk factors for cancer and other diseases.

So when dealing with larger medical conditions, be sure to explore all of your options and address the lifestyle pieces that you can before you choose medicine. In many cases, there are better choices that can keep the medications at bay and tip the energy scales in your favor.

Feeling better and alleviating one problem usually has a domino effect and leads to other benefits. Curing sleep apnea, for example, will infuse you with more energy because the body will be so happy to have continuous oxygen. This in turn will motivate you to get up in the morning and exercise, which has its own host of benefits that will come back to boost your health and energy. Remember, there's no magic bullet to managing or curing illness or dysfunction.

When was the last time you had a heart to heart with your doctor about your health and any medical conditions that you may be treating? If it's been a while since your last checkup, now is the time to schedule a new one. Take inventory of all your medications, vitamins, and supplements. Bring them with you and ask about how your daily doses could be affecting your energy levels, and if there are any alternatives to consider. You might be surprised to find that you don't really need to be taking some of your medication anymore, or that another, newer version of a certain drug has emerged on the market that has fewer side effects. Diagnosing and managing medical conditions often requires a team effort—you and your doctor, dietitian, trainer, therapist, and so on.

CHAPTER 7

Reboot:
Cleanse and Supplement

I feel pure and happy and much lighter.
I dropped the extra pounds that I had gained during a majorly fun
and delicious "relax-and-enjoy-life phase" about a month ago.

— G W Y N E T H   P A L T R O W ,
on her detox diet

Detox diets have gained popularity in the last few years, no doubt spurred by Hollywood's fixation on them like a sparkly accessory. But are they safe? Do they work? Which kind is best?

You may lose weight sipping lemon water with cayenne pepper for days, but radical fasting detoxes and master cleanses such as these, especially when done for rapid weight loss, can challenge the body much more than your current daily routine. They can deny your body of nutrients it needs, downshift your metabolism, and leave you more sensitive to foods, beverages, and your normal daily chaos when you return to your precleanse eating habits. Not to mention they are a metabolic recipe for energy loss. During a fast the body slows its systems and workload to compensate for a perceived lack of nutrients. To this end, if your cleanse doesn't supply sufficient nutrients (the range of nutrients—carbs, proteins, healthy fats) it's likely that the body may alter its metabolic functions in a way that prevents sustainable results and may compromise short-term energy and immune function. Not a good thing for your health or your energy.

For a true detox that will have lasting results, you needn't look further than the ideas already presented in this book. Eating a balanced, clean diet per the guidelines in Part II, coupled with adequate physical activity is more than enough to keep your body mean, lean, and clean—and does so without any of the side effects of an extreme detox. When people come to us for the secrets to detoxing the body, it usually means they've been indulging in their own "relax and enjoy life" phase of being less mindful of their dietary choices or they haven't been engaging in regular exercise and think a detox will help jump-start their efforts. They find themselves feeling low on energy and thicker around the waist thanks to eating lots of processed and classic junk food, and washing it down with enough wine to make a desperate housewife look good. What they really seek in a detox program is motivation to go back to basics and evict all the things that tax their body's optimal functioning.

In some instances, someone may ask about a detox program as they are recovering from treatments or battling with digestive or immune-related issues. They wonder if a detox will clear out whatever is disagreeing with their body. This is actually the worst time for a detox, as the body is in a weaker state and needs nutrient support. The body should be given the resources it requires to attend to its physiologic needs.

While the word *detoxification* may conjure images of drugged-out celebrities in rehab for substance abuse, from a scientific perspective it actually refers primarily to the body's natural methods of self-cleansing—of ridding waste that are the by-products of its normal function, and dealing with potentially harmful invaders such as bacteria, viruses, or toxic chemicals. Detoxification is a constant bodily process. We are continually eliminating excess toxins through our digestive, urinary, skin, circulatory, respiratory, and lymphatic systems and processes.

Rather than thinking of detoxification as a way of eliminating energy-depleting elements from your body, think of detoxification as a way of giving your body the equipment it needs to effectively act as its own shield against energy-depleting ingredients and incoming toxins, some of which we just cannot circumvent today. Detoxification helps fuel the engines that will literally clean up your body on a cellular level and support its natural operations. It also can physically re-boot your body so you can begin to make those small but transformational shifts in your lifestyle that will help you to live a more energetic life.

Earlier we paid homage to Dr. Mark Hyman's *UltraMetabolism*, in which he calls for detoxifying the liver as a critical step to weight loss, pointing to the fact a healthy functioning liver makes for a healthy functioning metabolism that can properly process sugars and fats. He underscores the fact that toxins from within our bodies and from our environment both contribute to obesity. So getting rid of toxins and boosting the natural detoxification system is an essential component of long-term weight loss and a healthy—energy-generating—metabolism.

We don't want to sound any alarms or scare you about the fact that we all live in a toxic world today. We have become a society where we no longer have to worry so much about things such as plague, famine, and poor sanitation. We now suffer from the products and by-products of our own technological advancements that provoke poor health and chronic illness. Myriad products we meet daily can harbor toxic substances that our bodies absorb little by little over time—from mattresses and mouthwash to carpets, clothing, and cosmetics.

And a lot resides in our food where preservatives, additives, coloring agents, pesticides, and other chemical residues hide. It's been argued that the reason fat cells bear the brunt of storing toxins is because our bodies were never designed to protect themselves from these toxins. So instead of the body being able to efficiently eliminate them, it throws them into fat cells much like you throw clutter in the garage or basement to deal with later. You're not quite sure what to do with it, so you store it somewhere that's out of sight (and temporarily out of mind). But as the toxins accumulate, they begin to have nasty effects on your body's functioning. You can begin to experience health problems, from minor ones such as allergies and endless colds, to serious illnesses such as cancer and brain disease. Lack of energy will be just the tip of the iceberg.

Skin Deep: Your skin is your largest organ. Keeping it healthy and red-carpet glowy goes way beyond the right facial or access to a cosmetic dermatologist. It begins at home—with a healthy digestive system, proper hydration, and regular exercise. The secrets to great-looking skin aren't all that secret by now. They originate in the diet:

- *Go Pro:* Add probiotics to your diet.

- *Animal Exchange:* Choose vegetarian fats and proteins rather than animal fats and proteins (e.g., scoop up nuts and seeds, and spread their oils and butters; and swap your steak for quinoa).

- *Don't Have a Cow:* Skip dairy in favor of healthy vegetarian sources of protein, such as quinoa and hemp seeds (e.g., pass on cheese, but pass the organic eggs). Or opt for organic dairy in limited amounts.

- *Get Green and Yellow:* Get your organic greens in several times daily to help with detoxification and use lemons and limes, which provide alkalinizing benefits in the digestive tract.

And any attempt at healthy skin must include a regular fitness routine that gets the circulation going, blood pumping, and your skin sweating. Try the following quick remedies for spot treatments:

- Slather the body with organic coconut oil after a shower.

- Dry-brush to improve lymphatic circulation and minimize cellulite (you can find dry-skin brushes at most beauty-supply stores).

- Stretch before and after your workout.

- Run with a sweatshirt on. Ever wonder how those got their name? They help to get you to sweat more if you wear them during your workout (Rocky Balboa style).

- Schedule a spa day with a friend and sit in the sauna and/or steam bath for a long, sweaty soak.

After all, who doesn't feel energized when they have great skin?

Another way to look at this is to consider what happens when the body tries to process toxins that the liver cannot easily break down. The toxins that are fat soluble will be sent to your fat cells, so the more toxins you have to store away, the more fat tissue your body needs to store them (and use precious energy to do so). And the fatter you become. This largely explains why detox programs ultimately help people to lose weight—and gain energy. Their body is able to release these stored toxins from the fat cells, rendering the fat cell empty.

They lose the need for the extra fat to begin with, and more energy can thus be conserved.

Avoiding the fat-soluble toxins may sound like a solution, but that's difficult to do today. We have considerable exposure to fat-soluble, carbon-containing, toxic chemicals used as solvents, glues, and paints. Common cleaning products, formaldehyde, toluene, and benzene are all solvents (meaning they are capable of dissolving other substances) we can typically encounter in daily life when we pump gas, shop for clothes, buy a new car, and pick up laundry. These fat-soluble chemicals collect in the fatty tissues of the body rather than being excreted quickly. They are particularly damaging to those who are deficient in essential fatty acids, because a body deprived of essential fats is a body that will grab on to oily substances—even if that includes toxic substances such as diesel fuel—similar to how a dry sponge readily soaks up water.

It's unrealistic to think we can totally eliminate all the potentially harmful substances in the world, their risk factors, and their energy-depleting effects. The best we can do is limit and manage our exposure—without driving ourselves crazy. If you've already begun to employ the ideas in the previous chapters, then you're well on your way to naturally detoxifying your system and making room for more energy. Adopting a healthy lifestyle for some people, though, is a challenge. It helps to go through a more specific protocol that sets the tone and gives you a much-needed launching pad.

Well, let this chapter be your starting point then. We're going to give you two step-by-step action plans for making our strategies come alive. Try either the 8-Day Deep Cleanse or the 3-Day Quick Cleanse and see how you feel. If you're really feeling ambitious, start with the 3-Day Cleanse and transition to the 8-Day Deep Cleanse. We bet you come out looking and feeling more energized, and it will show through your skin, too.

The 8-Day Deep Cleanse

This is about doing an energy-boosting cleanse that works with your body rather than against it. It's really simple: skip processed and packaged foods, chemicals, sugar, alcohol, and caffeine, and replace them with organic vegetables, whole grains, and healthy fats . . . and you've got yourself a cleanse that will work with the body. If you're (mostly) already doing this or looking for a jump start, you can also do a liquid cleanse of pureed organic vegetables, a little fruit, and vegetarian sources of protein, which will relax the body. (Because liquids don't require engaging the digestive process as much, the body can get to some of its deeper cleaning at this time.)

On each day, you must also engage in something physically demanding for at least 30 minutes. Examples: power walk in a hilly neighborhood, use a piece of gym equipment and spend time at an intensity that's slightly uncomfortable, attend a group class, perform at least five of the exercises showcased in the appendix, etc.

Note that you can choose to do all eight strategies at once starting on day one and continuing through all eight days. Or add one component at a time, one day after the other.

Day 1: Clean Up

Get rid of any packaged foods containing high-fructose corn syrup, hydrogenated oils, colors with pound signs (#) by them (e.g., blue lake #3), and artificial ingredients such as MSG (monosodium glutamate) or autolyzed yeast. You can have the kids help you out but be sure to check everything—you will be surprised what so-called healthy options may not be as healthy as they seem.

Day 2: Color Play

Aim to eat one serving of each of these colors (Skittles and Froot Loops don't count): red, blue, green, purple, and orange. Extra credit: choose organic (frozen organic is a great option).

Day 2 Hint: Stock your kitchen with colorful antioxidants. Plants offer the best source of antioxidants—the crusaders against free radicals. Eating up antioxidants will eat up those free radicals, preventing damage and ultimately boosting energy metabolism. While citrus fruits and berries are the most plentiful sources of antioxidants, all fruits and vegetables provide good supplies of antioxidants. The deeper and brighter the color of the food, the more densely packed with vitamins it is. Buy the most vividly colored fruits and veggies you can find. Make sure to keep some of the following all-star antioxidants in your kitchen as much as possible:

- Blueberries, raspberries, and strawberries

- Pomegranates, blackberries, and açai

- Vitamin A sources: carrots, mangoes

- Vitamin C sources: kiwis, mangoes, papayas, black currants, camu camu berries

- Vitamin E sources: nuts, seeds, whole grains, dark green leafy vegetables

Day 3: Some Assembly Required

Eat one to two (one for weight loss or if your physical activity is low) servings of carbohydrates and proteins, and one of healthy fat per eating occasion. Still hungry? Serve up some unlimited vegetables. Examples: apple + 1 tablespoon almond butter; palm-sized wild salmon + sauteed garlic spinach + fist-sized portion of rice; bowl of organic berries + drizzle of chocolate sauce.

Day 4: Beverage Patrol

Drink one cup of coffee or tea max for the day. For maximum metabolic and fat-burning advantages, go for green tea and oolong. Go decaf the rest of the day and no beverages with sugar—even if they promote their product as just a little sweet or no sugar added.

Day 4 Hint: Veto the vitamin water. Water isn't meant to be a source of vitamins. Yes, you need both vitamins and water, but not in a beverage with additives often including sugar; additionally, these vitamins aren't typically as easy for the body to use as the vitamins we get from quality food sources. Some water naturally contains minerals, but vitamins? Really? For the same grams of carbs in the water, you can eat a small banana, which is naturally rich in energy-revving B vitamins and potassium, and whose nutrients are likely much more bioavailable (ahem, easily absorbed).

Day 5: Treat Yourself

Remind yourself how great nonfood gifts can be to give and receive. Book a massage, get a manicure/pedicure, do something with a friend, or indulge in a long night out with your husband while the kids are well taken care of by a babysitter.

Day 6: Exchange—Part 1

Swap an animal for a vegetarian source of protein today. Ideas: organic nut butter on an apple. A veggie burger. Hemp granola or hemp seeds with a bowl of organic berries. Hummus and veggies. A bowl of quinoa with chopped walnuts, ground flaxseed, cinnamon, and ginger.

Day 6 Hint: For a list of AKA-approved brands, go to www.AshleyKoffRD.com.

Day 7: Exchange—Part 2

Swap high-fat dairy and less healthy animal fats for vegetarian sources (e.g., hemp, flax, olive, avocado, coconut) and wild fish (e.g., sardines, cod, salmon), or choose organic lower fat dairy options including goat and sheep sources. Try different cultured veggies or tempeh. Exchanging organic and antibiotic-free dairy as well as adding fermented foods will decrease antibiotics and increase probiotics.

Day 7 Hint: For a list of AKA-approved brands, go to www.AshleyKoffRD.com.

Day 8: Flavor from Nature

Spice up your cooking by using cardamom, oregano, thyme, ginger, cinnamon, and fennel seeds.

ASHLEY'S ENERGY ADVICE

I recently had a *Shedding for the Wedding* cast member ask me after months of massive changes and the resulting weight loss and health gains, "Do I need a cleanse?" And I said, "My dear, you've been on a cleanse for months—no sodas, no artificial ingredients, lots of exercise, lots of veggies, super good quality foods, not much red meat, etc. . . ." Skip the packaged deal you saw at the market and stay the course!

THE 3-DAY QUICK CLEANSE

For those who need to be handheld through a quick cleanse, try the following 12-step program every day for three full days.

1. On waking, take a probiotic with hot tea or hot water with lemon.

2. Stretch, do some exercise. You may feel hungry or slightly lightheaded so adjust your pace/duration accordingly but even 15 minutes will net some fat-burning effects.

3. Make a protein-greens drink with water (or coconut water) and a healthy fat like avocado. See www.AshleyKoffRD.com for brand ideas and recipes. Drink slowly and take a vitamin D_3 supplement.

4. Sip on hot beverages (herbal tea, water with lemon) throughout the morning. If starving, add almond or rice milk (organic, plain).

5. Midmorning: have a snack of 1 cup organic applesauce and 1 tablespoon flaxseeds or chia seeds.

6. Midday: this is your best time for an eating occasion. Try organic veggies or veggie soup (pureed, no dairy) with vinegars or hempseeds, herbs, and spices. Roasted and sautéed veggies are great too if done with a healthy organic oil.

7. Midafternoon: perhaps a self-made tea latte, unless you have a place that does organic almond or rice milk and *no* sweetener. Most commercial coffee shops making tea lattes use both sugar-based tea powders and sweeteners or sweetened soy milk, so make sure you ask. Add some veggies or cultured veggies with hemp seeds, spices, and dressing, or a small cup of soup or real seaweed salad (not the neon green sweet one at the store). If you're not into all the "fancy stuff," cut up some cucumber, jicama, and celery and mix it with cayenne and lime to make a great crunchy snack option.

8. Before 7 P.M.: blend up a smoothie but skip the added greens if you have trouble sleeping.

Note: all of these eating occasions are interchangeable, so if you go out to dinner, get an organic greens salad and soup (maybe bring your hemp seeds or dressing or just opt for lemon juice). Or if you have a morning meeting, have your drink and get sautéed veggies at the meeting.

9. About 1 hour before bed take a magnesium citrate supplement that aids sleep and stress reduction. (Magnesium citrate prodcuts are available as an organic powdered form.) Dosage should reflect your regularity—if you are having regular bowel movements go with 1 to 2 teaspoons.

10. Consider dry brushing the skin, a hot bath or shower, coconut oil on wet skin, a facial mask for 20 minutes, and using a roller to roll out your muscles.

11. If you can, during the cleanse wear minimal or no makeup or nail polish and let the body air itself out.

12. Get regular exercise (yes, you want to sweat), schedule a massage and infrared sauna sessions, practice yoga, take long (hilly!) walks, and find time to sit in silence.

EXIT GRACEFULLY

When followed properly, a quality cleanse can work effectively to help us shift seasons, to get out of a mental or physical fog, or to jump-start weight-loss goals and live a more health-conscious life.

You want to ease your body back into a healthier diet. Start by eating foods easily digested, such as lightly cooked vegetables. Then move to fruit and whole grains. Pay attention to portion control and frequency of eating occasions. Eat vegetable protein before animal protein, and avoid known gastric irritants. Continue to consume water and liquids for hydration. Keep a food-mood journal and notice how a reintroduction of certain foods makes you feel. If you had given something up, assess why you feel you need to return to it. For example, if you were used to drinking a glass of wine nightly or coffee at your break, what has it been like to avoid that? This doesn't mean you can't have it, but it helps to look at the why. And be sure to get your rest. You may be done with the cleanse, but your body is working through changes. Let it.

Supplement Smartly

With so many supplements on the market today, one frequently asked question is does the form of the vitamin—tablet, capsule, liquid, powder, spray—matter? YES! And is there a particular set of supplements you should be taking? YES! You have to supplement smartly.

The type of nutrient in a supplement matters a great deal—for example, d-alpha tocopherol (as a vitamin E source) is not identical to dl-alpha tocopherol. That one extra letter spells the difference between natural and synthetic, as in nut versus photo paper. Yup, you read that right—photo paper! And what about magnesium oxide versus magnesium citrate? There is a major difference in absorption. And oftentimes minerals—not necessarily vitamins—can be a much bigger issue when it comes to optimizing energy.

Even the best, healthiest eater can benefit from supplements today. It's simply a fact of life given our habits and stress levels (both of which can strip our bodies of nutrients). Certain health challenges can also be a factor. If you've recently had surgery, take medication on a regular basis, or are in the throes of menopause—these can change your body's needs and supplies of the ingredients it requires to run like a champion. If you've ever had problems with digestion after taking supplements, try taking them in the middle of a meal. Never take supplements on an empty stomach unless instructed to do so by your doctor. Following are some more guidelines to consider:

Multivitamin and mineral supplement. Remember the movie *Jerry Maguire*? In one of the movie's most memorable scenes, Tom Cruise's character says to Renée Zellweger's character, "You complete me." That's exactly what you're going for when it comes to taking a daily multivitamin. Even if you eat well, you're bound to run low on a few nutrients due to the realities of life (hey, no one can eat perfectly all the time). So select a comprehensive and balanced formula containing all the major vitamins, minerals, and trace minerals; select an iron-free formula if you are postmenopausal. Look for high-quality, organic forms of the ingredients. For example, the fact that vitamin E works at the mitochondrial rather than cellular level, and does not work at the blood level, is proof that synthetic vitamin E ("dl-alpha tocopherol") is an ineffective form; you'll want to take d-alpha tocopherol, which is vitamin E in its natural form. Ideally, go for gluten-free; and if you've got a history of digestive issues, try a food-based liquid vitamin to ensure bioavailability of nutrients and optimal absorption.

Magnesium. Make sure that you are getting sufficient magnesium to counterbalance supplemental and food intake of calcium. Seek a magnesium citrate supplement, which will absorb better than magnesium oxide. Magnesium creates the calm—whether it's mental or physical; it turns off our stress response, allows our muscles to relax (which means all muscles: especially our digestive tract muscles), and is critical for strong bones along with its partner calcium. Magnesium is responsible for more than 300 metabolic reactions in our body, and it's thought that over 50 percent of the U.S. population is deficient in magnesium. Our current decline in adequate magnesium is partly due to a combination of food processing (white flour has 60 to 80 percent less magnesium than whole-wheat grain), an avoidance of magnesium-rich carbs in general, and a decrease of this mineral in our soils due to chemical farming versus organic. Magnesium-rich foods include whole grains, artichoke, beans, nuts and seeds, dark leafy greens, and even some chocolate. It's practically pointless to get plenty of calcium if you're not getting your magnesium as well, because they work in tandem.

B Complex. You'll find plenty of B vitamins in a variety of foods (chiefly brewer's yeast, wheat germ, whole grains, beans, dark green vegetables, low-fat and nonfat dairy, fish, eggs, and poultry), but to ensure that you get an adequate daily supply, it's best to supplement with a B complex every day that covers all eight Bs—thiamine (B_1), riboflavin (B_2), niacin (B_3), pantothenic acid (B_5), pyridoxine (B_6), biotin (B_7), folic acid (B_9), and cyanocobalamin (B_{12}). These gems are important to energy metabolism and can easily be stripped from the body as a result of stress and certain medicines. Women who take the birth-control pill, for example, have been shown to have low blood levels of B vitamins, which may then trigger migraines.

Essential fatty acid supplements. There are certain fatty acids (omega-3s and -6s) that the body doesn't make, so it's necessary that we get these from the food we eat. Like our multivitamins, which provide foundational support for vitamins and minerals, essential fatty acid supplements can provide these nutrients to ensure we meet our required daily intake. For optimal energy and health, we recommend dietary supplements from whole food forms. This may be in the form of fish oil (especially from wild salmon), flaxseed, chia, and hempseed oils. Vegetarians or those not eating fish or taking fish oil supplements can also choose micro-algae-derived DHA and EPA supplements. Shoot for at least 500 mg of omega-3.

Supplements for bone health. While recommendations used to be for just calcium, we know today that bone health requires a mixture of nutrients including vitamins D and K and minerals like calcium and magnesium, as well as other trace minerals. An evaluation of your diet, your bone-building efforts, and any bone health risks with your doctor can help determine the best supplementation plan for you to achieve your healthy-bone goal.

Vitamin D. Vitamin D has gained a lot of attention in recent years due to an enormous body of research confirming its role in human health and the fact that we don't get enough of it. It's not just a result of us working indoors all day and protecting ourselves from the sun's damaging rays, but it's also a consequence of geography. The vast majority of people who live in North America can't get the same amount of sunlight as those closer to the equator. It's easy for the body to manufacture plenty of vitamin D from brief exposure to UVB radiation a few times a week, but it's very hard to get that same amount of vitamin D from diet alone. Why is this vitamin so important? It's actually a hormone critical to survival because it has a role in numerous communications. A number of studies have found that higher vitamin D, which the body makes when sunlight hits the skin, protects against some cancers and illnesses such as rickets, bone-thinning osteoporosis, and diabetes. It also helps the body's immune system work properly; reduces inflammation; and plays a role in muscle, cardiac, immune, and neurological functions. If you're not casually exposed to sunlight for brief periods a few days a week ("brief" meaning 10 to 15 minutes and long before you'd begin to burn), consider adding a vitamin D supplement that has at least 1,000 IU to your daily regimen.

Antioxidants. If your multivitamin also contains a blend of antioxidants, more power to you. In addition to the usual suspects (vitamins A, C, E), you might also find others, such as alpha lipoic acid, citrus bioflavonoids, extracts from teas and grapes, milk thistle, n-acetyl cysteine, quercetin, curcumin (turmeric), selenium, and coenzyme Q10. Note: While some antioxidants have a recommended daily allowance, such as vitamins A, C, and E, most do not. Instead of trying to count milligrams of your antioxidant intake, just try to get as many of these into your diet from colorful organic fruits and vegetables as possible.

Iron alert. Before you consider supplementing iron, get tested for iron-deficiency anemia. You don't want excess iron in your system, especially post-menopausal women who don't lose iron through blood loss regularly, as excess iron can function as an unwanted prooxidant (the opposite of antioxidant). Additionally, iron supplementation can cause or exacerbate constipation. That said, if you're still in your reproductive years and menstruate regularly, you lose iron each month. Unless it's replaced in your diet or with the combination of diet and supplements, you could suffer some of the unpleasant symptoms of iron-deficiency anemia—chronic exhaustion being one of them.

STAYING TRUE TO FORM

If you're on a diet or detoxing, what do your children think when you don't eat with them at the table or nibble on something strange that they'd never eat? What kind of messages are you giving them? Staying true to yourself and your role as mom is critical.

Many of you don't really start to think about yourself as a "role model" until your children are conscious of you and your habits. That's when it becomes imperative to pay closer attention to your actions. If you don't eat like your kids, what message are you sending? Kids learn through watching and attempting to mimic their parents. Think about where you learned your habits—both good and bad. Remember, your kids are watching you as much or more than they are listening to you. Don't expect your child to love being active if you're not. If they ask where you are going and you say, "I have to go work out; I have to use my muscles," they will begin to understand the importance of exercise. They need to know that you spent part of your day in a workout.

The same holds true with eating. Let them be curious and ask questions about your diet choices. If you eat a salad with the dressing on the side, share with them why it's much easier to control how much unhealthy fat you're consuming so you can ultimately have more energy for them. When you're enjoying a side of French fries with your broccoli and chicken, you can discuss balance. Teach them the difference between an occasional treat and unlimited indulgence. Most moms want to demonstrate a healthy and active lifestyle for kids; it sets them up for a lifetime of healthy habits. This message should also ring loud and clear for grandmothers, too. It's common for grandmothers to indulge grandchildren with treats and splurges. But grandmothers can set good examples as much as mothers can by cooking healthy meals and engaging in physical activities with their grandchildren. Parents who eat differently than their kids can unwittingly do damage that can then be difficult to change. For example, picture the mom who orders a salad while her kids get the Whopper. Or she eats a Lean Cuisine and orders a pizza for her kids. Given the rising rates of obesity among children today, we need to rethink how we fuel our families. Similarly, if mom goes to an exercise class while the kids stay home and watch TV or play video games, this pattern over time can spell trouble. Think about ways in which you can include all of your family members in your whole journey and mission to be a healthy, energetic mother. Otherwise, your life will backfire and the challenges that surface will do nothing but take away your energy and any hope of recovering it. Besides, to be a fully engaged mother and feel fulfilled in your role, it helps to participate in your kids' lives as much as possible—at the table, on the playing field, and in their day-to-day choices. Kids will eat what's put in front of them. They will copy a parent who shows enthusiasm for regular exercise. They will come to admire the fact that you make healthy choices to maximize your energy reserves for their benefit.

Something else to keep in mind: marketers would have you believe that kids should eat separately. They'd like nothing more than to encourage you to buy two types of dinners—one for your kids and another for you. It shouldn't be that way. If the kids are having chicken fingers, then so should you. It bears repeating: Bring your kids into the conversation about health early. Let them help you decide what you're having for dinner as a family. Remember, you're teaching a lifestyle. There's nothing more unappealing than an adult who doesn't eat vegetables and whose favorite food is chicken fingers, mac and cheese, and pizza. You're not a parent on some days of the week or during certain hours of the day. You're a parent 24/7, so be a role model every minute of the day as well. Let that responsibility inform all of your decisions and your kids will love you for it. Being true to form all the time is what will allow you to really maximize your entire energetic life. As this next part shows, you'll optimize your time, capitalize on your sleep, and make the most out of the stressors that compete with your energy.

MOM UP! JUMP-START YOUR TRANSFORMATION

If the thought of removing certain foods to do a detox as outlined in this chapter just isn't your thing, then start by slowly adding the supplements that were discussed. If you don't already take a multivitamin, start with this. Go to your local health-food store and ask about which brands are recommended. Whole Foods, for example, has its own "whole body" section with a designated person there who is well versed in all the varieties they sell. If you already take a multivitamin daily but nothing else, then aim to add another supplement or two to your daily regimen. Soon you'll be getting just what you need to fill in any blanks. Bring a list based on the guidelines we've given and ask the store representative for help in purchasing the highest-quality supplements possible for you. (Alternatively, you can visit our websites at www.kathykaehler.net and www.AshleyKoffRD.com for our own lists of brands we recommend.)

PART IV

RECHARGE

CHAPTER 8

Make Magic
with Movement:
Bring Exercise into Your Day

Positivity is energy. Always leave the party when you are having fun.
And when I can remember to count my blessings,
balance is naturally restored.

— SARAH SCHLEPER DE GAXIOLA,
Olympic skier, mother

Julia Roberts perhaps said it best when she declared, "Don't tell me I look tired. Just tell me I look like a mom!"

When moviegoers watched a ravishing Julia emerge bikini-clad out of a swimming pool in the 2007 movie *Charlie Wilson's War*, women everywhere wondered how she did it at four months pregnant with twins. Later, for her role in *Eat Pray Love*, Julia focused her attention again on getting in shape to handle the rigors of moviemaking, which took place around the world and back as she juggled three kids under age ten. At the film's New York premiere, she was photographed on the red carpet wearing a feminine tuxedo in short shorts. Her long, toned legs looked endless. Once more, the questions circled: How did she get those legs? What does she do?

To the dismay of some moms, who wish the secret were a new trick they hadn't heard of yet, Julia's secret weapon was none less than a classic step workout. It may scream circa 1990, but it worked magic and could be used just about anywhere. She'd go up and down on it for 40 minutes and mix her workouts up with other beloved traditions such as yoga and running. If there's anything "unusual" about her step workouts, though, it's that she often adds a friend to the routine. Even at the crack of dawn she'd make it fun by inviting someone to join her so they could talk and kill the time with laughter, movement, and a sharing of ideas. The topics would run the gamut, from better ways to recycle, recipes, and the kids' sleep habits, to gossip. Though a slight departure from what most people would call a "workout," it's a workout nonetheless. And with obvious results.

The moral of this story is that you don't have to close everything off and focus on just the exercise to get a fat-defying, energizing workout. Most moms can agree that exercise has to fit into your life and the business of your household. Granted, Julia has always been good at consistency, which is another key to keeping the body up to speed and which can be a challenge for moms who aren't exacting with their priorities and schedules. But of all the "secrets" we hear about when it comes to sculpting the body and maintaining fitness, we often don't think about the bonus of nurturing friendships at the same time. Julia can't get sick of her workouts if she's simultaneously chatting with a friend and connecting with another mother. As women, we have an innate need to identify with other women, especially moms who share the same struggles of raising children. And for Julia, her workouts can be as much about the mental therapy of good conversation as they are about the body therapy of good exercise. It's as easy as that.

Here's something else to consider: Most of us ache to engage in lively, engrossing conversations. We rarely get the opportunity given the time constraints of motherhood and the dynamics of a typical day. Most of us have highly fragmented days—our minds are ricocheting from one crisis or commitment to the next faster than we are simultaneously transporting ourselves (and our brood) from one place to another. It's a recipe for energy loss. A mother's life does not dovetail the way we are designed to converse with other human beings where one topic is allowed to flow seamlessly into the next. When's the last time you engaged in an endless stream of thoughts with an old friend without having to think or worry about anything else? Imagine how that experience would add up to a big infusion of stress-relieving energy.

We're not saying that you have to exercise with friends every day, but the point is clear: it helps to view exercise as an opportunity to tune out your "real" world as an overscheduled mother and just be in the moment with your body. It's where you are allowed to finish a sentence. It's where you give yourself permission to have no interruptions and to focus on just yourself and perhaps another human being. Your body may be working hard, but your mind is relaxed. You don't feel exasperated. There's nothing more energy-building than that. Far too often we see women treat exercise as yet another chore, another To Do. It's boring. It's hard. It's exhausting. It's not fun, but it doesn't have to be that way. Far from it!

The message here isn't so much about what Julia does specifically to stay in shape, because any activity that gets you moving and your heart beating is enough to do the job. But it's how she goes about her activity that makes a difference. With the goal of losing herself among thoughts, friends, and a body in sweaty motion, she gets results that go farther than a nice pair of legs, or set of abs, or whatever. And that's probably the ultimate key to success in staying active and fit. Without that component you won't be motivated to do anything.

Profile Alert! All the profile types can benefit from the recommendations and information in this chapter. Whether you're The Medicine Cabinet (Profile 1), The Mom Zombie (Profile 2), The Overworked and Overscheduled (and Overtired) (Profile 3), The Chronic Dieter (Profile 4), or The Dead Battery (Profile 5), finding movement in your day is key to your well-being.

We usually think of exercise as leading to fatigue but a significant body of evidence shows that the immediate effect of exercise is increased energy. You've probably heard the mantra about exercise being good for you many times before (even in this book). But if there's one magic bullet for enhancing your energy and the amount you can keep on reserve, not to mention boost your looks, your mood, and your life in general, it's exercise. The science is well documented: exercise fights the onset of age-related disease, promotes a positive sense of well-being, increases your lung capacity so you can take in more oxygen, boosts circulation to deliver nutrients to cells, lowers inflammation, and for many is said to be the ultimate stress reducer.

Physically and mentally, exercise has profound effects on the body. All the intertwined biochemical activities that accompany exercise, from the release of anti-inflammatory endorphins that counteract the stress hormone cortisol to the increased circulation and deeper breathing, are a recipe for stress reduction and energy creation. That healthy glow you get after a great workout (rosy cheeks indicative of the increased circulation that is nourishing all those facial cells and tissues) isn't just for show.

As we stated in the first chapter, the more lean muscle mass you have, and the more oxygen you can deliver to your body's tissues, the bigger your battery is. It's as simple as that. These two critical goals—more lean muscle mass and increased capacity to deliver oxygen throughout the body—are achieved through regular exercise. Recall, too, what we said about your most important energy packagers in the body: your mitochondria. The majority of the functions of mitochondria are to convert the energy in food into ATP—the molecule that provides energy for physiological processes. It's your body's energy currency.

The age and efficiency of your mitochondria have a direct correlation with your metabolic health. Because they are a center of gravity for your physiology, they are direct targets for cellular damage. Think about it: they charge your physiology but in doing so expose themselves to your physiology's by-products, including

Working the body physically lights up the energy powers from within, and sweating is physical evidence that you're powering up your battery. Do we need to remind you about the advantages of exercise that have long been reported and proven? All of the following benefits circle back to having a positive influence on your energy and the ability to sustain an optimal metabolism:

- Increased stamina

- Increased flexibility

- Increased blood circulation

- Increased oxygen supply to cells and tissues

- More restful, sound sleep

- Decreased stress

- Increased self-esteem and sense of well-being

- Increased muscle strength, tone, and endurance

- Increased levels of brain chemicals called endorphins that act as natural mood lifters and pain relievers

- Decreased food cravings

- Decreased blood-sugar levels, and risk for diabetes

- Improved weight distribution and maintenance

those pesky free radicals that can inflict harm and clog the very system designed to create and sustain your energy. In fact, the specialized energy conversion functions that the mitochondria perform make them and their DNA more susceptible to mutation than the normal DNA of the cell, which lies protected inside the nucleus of most cells. Those nasty free radicals will unwittingly attack the mitochondrial membranes and DNA—making them less efficient over time. For this reason, mitochondria have been called the Achilles' heel of the cell in aging.

And here's where we bring in the beauty about exercise. No doubt what you eat and what you expose yourself to in your environment affects the extent to which your mitochondria function and how much damage they endure, but people forget the influence that exercise has in this regard. Moderate intensity aerobic exercise for just 15 to 20 minutes, three to four times a week has been shown to increase the number of mitochondria in your muscle cells by 40 to 50 percent. That's not very much exercise for a huge increase in your energy metabolism (and ability to burn fat).

PUTTING THE ENERGY IN EXERCISE

Exercise physiology has come a long way in the last 20 years. We know so much more about the mechanics of the human body through laboratory and clinical tests that show us exactly what's going on when we decide to charge up a hill or train for a marathon. Entire new fields of medicine have been created, such as metabolomics, which is a form of metabolic profiling that aims to find patterns in people that either spell disease or lower their risk for certain illnesses. Out of this new field has come the confirmation that the fitter you are, the more benefit for your metabolism. This is due to metabolic changes that occur during exercise. In a study done by a team from Mass General, the Broad Institute of MIT, and Harvard, fit people were found to have greater increases in a metabolite called niacinamide than unfit people. Niacinamide is a nutrient by-product that's involved with blood-sugar control. In fact, this team found more than 20 metabolites that change during exercise. These are naturally produced compounds involved in burning calories and fat, and improving blood-sugar control. Some weren't known until now to be involved with exercise. Some revved up during exercise, such as those involved in processing fat. Others involved with cellular stress decreased with exercise.

Another recent discovery relates to the classic "runner's high"—the state of euphoria associated with prolonged exercise (talk about high energy!). It's no longer explained solely by the adrenaline and endorphin hypothesis. Scientists now believe that the physical and psychological well-being experienced by many endurance athletes is due to the exercise-induced activation of cannabinoids—lipids, in fact—in the body whose actions resemble those of the active ingredients of marijuana. These cannabinoids can suppress pain; they inhibit swelling and inflammation; and dilate blood vessels and make breathing easier. The phenomenon of exercise addiction is largely due to these powerful chemicals naturally produced in the body.

There's no end to the number of studies that prove the energy connection in relation to exercise. In 2009 another study emerged clearly showing that exercise causes your brain to turn up production of certain brain chemicals known to have antidepressant effects. Anything that helps us stave off depression and lift our spirits is good for energy. The researchers also found that exercise excited a gene for a nerve growth factor called VGF. VGFs are small proteins critical to the development and maintenance of nerve cells. Even more fascinating is the fact the study brought to light 33 VGFs that show altered activity with exercise, the majority of which had never been identified before.

With all this new information, there's been plenty of confusing and seemingly conflicting data. It's been proven, for example, that just 10 minutes of brisk walking (now that's low-tech!) enhances energy levels for up to 90 minutes thereafter. This is partly due to the discoveries just made about exercise triggering metabolic changes that last at least an hour—especially for those who are already in shape. But this isn't enough to keep us in shape. It's also been shown that moderate exercise at least five days a week for 30 minutes a pop will not result in long-term weight loss and maintenance. So how do we rectify all the competing information?

If you work out for an hour at a moderate level, you will burn and recharge only so much depending on where you are physically. Many people casually work on the StairMaster or the elliptical, for example, and count the minutes as they go by just to say, "I did 30 minutes today." When they complain of not getting the results they want, we have to remind them that their battery demands to be challenged in the exercise department. You can't just move more in daily life; you have to up the ante. This entails going hard in a workout a few days a week to stress your aerobic capacity and to put pressure on your bones so they are forced to stay strong. It could mean the difference between looking okay but not feeling great.

People forget the effects that aging has on the body and the ability to maintain a strong energy metabolism. In addition to the muscle loss and strength that we experience naturally alongside the inevitable slowdown of our metabolisms over time, we fail to consider the practical reasons for weight gain and energy depletion: we have a tendency to become more sedentary yet don't change our eating habits. Hormonal changes put more nails in the coffin, exacerbating an already troubled energy metabolism. This is why a study released in 2010 and published in the *Journal of the American Medical Association* stated clearly that the 2008 U.S. guidelines urging about a half hour of exercise five days a week won't stop weight gain while getting older without cutting calories. Put another way, it takes more to lose more as you age more. According to this latest study, older women at a healthy weight need to engage in moderate activity for at least an hour a day if they want to maintain their weight without changing their diets. The research is more sobering for those who are already overweight: even more exercise is called for to avoid gaining weight without eating less.

KATHY'S ENERGY ADVICE

Since hitting the onset of menopause, I've had to seriously crank up the intensity of my workouts. I went through a year of being achy, feeling bad, and gaining weight no matter what I did. My body was in a standstill. One day, exasperated but determined to find something that worked, I decided to test the limits of my physicality and charge up a hill on my mountain bike like a madwoman. It shocked my system, but it's exactly what I needed. I had to get my heart rate up so high that my body was forced to respond. Since then, everything has changed. I feel far more in control now. I have this energy that's very reliable. Rather than feed my body excuses like "I can't get out of bed," I remind myself that I can rise at 5 A.M., I can do 17 loads of laundry (if I need to!), and I no longer spend hours at night facing racing thoughts and anxiety. I sleep like a baby.

Reaching the inevitable hormonal shifts had its hidden benefits. It compelled me to stop and think about the choices I was making. It demanded that I go back to basics—to really look at calorie expenditure and how hard I was pushing myself physically. For me, that meant finding an activity that burns hundreds of calories and gets me outside. It's imperative for you to have something that allows you to jack up that heart rate, cover yourself in sweat, and reach a point where you're panting. Right away, you'll feel this rush of "Oh my gosh!" That's your energy tap. Open that up. Foods do play a huge role, but the physical part of exercise is also where it's at. Think of it this way: We're not churning the butter. We're not putting our clothes on the line, washing our cars, or doing any physical labor like we used to. You've got to do something else if you don't want to take this other route of reluctantly succumbing to changes in your body. Walk or bike ride up a steep hill, or climb stadium stairs. Get a trainer to make you work out harder. Find a friend who is more fit than you and tag along. Make goals for yourself. Don't let the excuses pile on. You can find something!

The Fountain of Youth

Energy is often equated with youth. When you're young, you have more energy, feel more energetic, and look the part, too. This isn't just a sensation. Our age can be seen in our genes, and we can also see the difference that physical activity makes.

The idea that exercise can "reverse" aging is no longer proven by anecdotal evidence alone. It's been an area of intense and exciting research worldwide. In 2008, for example, a team of Canadian and American researchers showed that exercise can partially help reverse the aging process at the cellular level. They looked at the effects of six months of strength training in elderly volunteers aged 65 and older. They took small biopsies of thigh-muscle cells from the seniors before and after the six-month period, then compared them with muscle cells from 26 young volunteers whose average age was 22. The scientists expected to find evidence that the program improved the seniors' strength, which it did by 50 percent. But they never expected what else they witnessed: dramatic changes at the genetic level. The genetic fingerprint of those elderly volunteers who'd gone through the strength-training program was reversed nearly to that of younger people. In other words, their genetic profile resembled that of a younger group.

How did they measure this change and difference? At the beginning of the six-month period, researchers found significant differences between the older and younger participants in the expression of 600 genes, indicating that these genes become either more or less active with age. By the end of the exercise phase, the expression of a third of those genes had changed, and upon closer observation they realized that the ones that changed were the genes involved in the functioning of mitochondria. That's right: it all goes back to your mitochondria, your cells' chief generators where ATP gets created to process nutrients into energy.

Giving you a detailed exercise program is not the goal of this chapter. Instead, we're going to present a few ideas to consider in pursuit of establishing your own unique routine. The goal is to inspire exercise for energy, and to show how the "what we do" becomes the "how much E we have" in the day. Put another way, when you know how to find the right balance of testing and respecting your body's limits from a physical standpoint, you can achieve that Holy Grail of optimizing your energy.

(For those dying for a list of best exercises you can do just about anywhere, we invite you to flip to the appendix. There, you'll find The Whole-Body List that includes basic step-by-step instructions.

THE ESSENTIALS TO THE ENERGY EQUATION

The type of activity you do is not nearly as important as how often you do it and how long you do it. Because exercise lowers stress for up to 24 hours, it's important to avoid being the "weekend warrior" and make it a goal of keeping a semi-daily routine. Remember, consistency is key. It's also critical that you match your body to where it's at physically, and even emotionally. If it's having to use its resources elsewhere, say to fight a cold or breastfeed a baby, then your personal exercise program won't be the same as someone else's. One great question to ask yourself is: What exercise will address what my mind and body need? If you are mad at work, for example, you may need to work it out aggressively on a hard run or dance class so you don't take that negative energy home. But if your kid was up sick all night and you got little sleep, you may just need a simple walk and a nap.

Ultimately, we want to make sure that we don't ask too much of the body, while at the same time encourage it to test its limits once in a while in order to get stronger and build endurance—the kind of endurance every mother needs.

When Angie Harmon tried to get back into shape for a new series after having her third child, she still looked fabulous. But her physical shape told a different story in the gym. Angie battled serious back problems stemming from the pregnancy that traveled down to her legs, for which lots of stretch-and-hold exercises (for 30 to 60 seconds) came to the rescue. To boost her endurance, which also had hit an all-time low, cardio and weight training helped get her back into the game.

Ideally, a well-rounded and comprehensive exercise program that optimizes your energy metabolism includes cardio work, strength training, and stretching. Each of these activities affords you unique benefits that your body needs to achieve and maintain peak performance. Cardio work, which gets your heart rate up for an extended period of time, will burn calories, lower body fat, and strengthen both your heart and lungs. Strength training (use of weights or elastic bands, or even your own body weight as resistance in some cases) will keep your bones strong and prevent that loss of lean muscle mass. Stretching will keep you flexible and less susceptible to joint pain.

Also don't forget that the benefits of exercise are cumulative. Another fact science has proven is that short exercise bouts throughout the day are just as effective as one long workout and may be even better. So you don't have to sweat it out on a treadmill for a full 60 minutes all in a row. You can do 10 minutes here, 20 minutes there. The reason for this is twofold. First, interval training that really gets your heart and lungs thumping trumps the slow-and-steady exercise routine. The essence of interval training is going hard for a short period of time, then backing off for a few minutes before resuming a higher level of intensity again for another short interval. You can do this in virtually any type of exercise, from walking to utilizing equipment in a gym. Varying your speed, adding weights, or increasing the incline on, say, a walk outdoors on hills, are all ways in which you can create your own interval-training routine. Those bursts of high-intensity intervals will equate with bursts of high-intensity energy! If you're not the type to zone out for an hour in a workout like Julia Roberts, then sprinkle pockets of workout times into your day—at lunch, after dinner, or in the 15 minutes right after you get up and the house is still quiet.

Consistency can be too idealistic. Life with kids is dynamic, sporadic, and ever changing. Understand what your possibilities are. If you really want to work out, you have to take advantage of when you know you have the opportunities. When kids are napping or at school, seize the moment and do it. But if it gets away from you, there might be another window that could open up later on that you did not anticipate. We can't feel like if we miss a workout, it's the end of the world. Just shut down earlier and wake up earlier the next day to get it done. Sleep in workout clothes or have them next to the bed. Accept that you won't get it done and it's okay, but use that energy to plan the next day.

— ANGIE HARMON,
actress and mother of three

Cut to the Chase

The second explanation behind the benefits of "burst" activity—spreading your workouts throughout the day into short bursts—is that it helps prevent you from the ravages that sitting down all day can do to you. We hope you're not sitting down while reading this. No joke: as we were putting together our materials for this book, researchers at the American Cancer Society released a study published in the *American Journal of Epidemiology* that pretty much said sitting down for extended periods poses a health risk as insidious as smoking or overexposure to the sun. A second study at the International Diabetes Institute in Melbourne concluded that even two hours of exercise a day would not compensate for "spending 22 hours sitting on your rear end."

While several studies support a link between sitting time and obesity, type 2 diabetes, risk factors for cardiovascular disease, and unhealthy dietary patterns in children and adults, very few studies have examined time spent sitting in relation to total mortality. This latest study makes a stunning case for the strong association between continually sitting down (as many of us do nowadays at desks, on the couch, and in our cars) and disease. The shocker: women seem to be more affected by spending time on their derrieres. In the study, women who reported more than six hours per day of sitting (outside of work) were 37 percent more likely to die during the time period studied than those who sat fewer than three hours a day. Men who sat more than six hours a day (also outside of work) were 18 percent more likely to die than those who sat fewer than three hours per day. The association remained virtually unchanged after adjusting for physical-activity level. The people in the study were followed from 1993 to 2006; researchers examined the participants' amount of time spent sitting and physical activity in relation to mortality over the 13-year period.

The act of sitting itself is not the culprit here. It's the biological effects that sitting triggers in the body that are a game changer. And by that we mean sitting's metabolic impact. Prolonged time spent sitting, independent of physical activity, has been shown to have significant metabolic consequences, negatively influencing levels of things such as triglycerides, high-density lipoprotein (the "good" cholesterol), blood sugar, resting blood pressure, and the appetite hormone leptin, all of which are biomarkers of obesity and cardiovascular and other chronic diseases.

The message is clear: you must move—and move frequently—to maintain health. It's not just a matter of energy. It's a matter of life and longevity. Even people who just break up their sitting time by walking to a friend's house rather than e-mailing her, for instance, have a lower risk of diabetes.

Whether it's a structured class at a gym, power walking with friends in the morning, dancing, or renting DVDs with the latest from fitness trainers, there are lots of options today. Get creative and have fun with your activity. Don't make it a chore, and don't make yourself miserable by doing something you hate.

Exercise should be enjoyable, something you look forward to every day. And remember, many forms of exercise can involve

What exercises can I do with my kids? I get this question a lot, because traditional forms of exercise typically exclude children unless you're playing with them in the park or at a jungle gym. However, there are lots of things you can do to engage your kids in a workout that has the added benefit of demonstrating to them the importance of leading a physically active life and making exercise a priority. You can also begin to teach them about taking care of their bodies and making them strong and fit.

The first thing I like to recommend is letting your kids do a workout DVD with you. They love to copy Mom—it makes them feel grown-up. Then I remind moms to take active vacations and schedule active family nights where you plan to do something physical together like bowl, go to the batting cages, dance, play Frisbee at the park, or just walk the dog after dinner. Finally, you might want to check out the use of a trampoline, which is not something just for kids. I've used these with Jennifer Lopez as well as Kim Basinger. Kim bought one for her daughter but then realized from my workout that it's a great way to get your heart rate up. You can play all kinds of games with your kids using a small trampoline that will fit in most dens or living rooms. Take turns jumping on it and challenge each other with how many jumps you can make with your toes pointed, tucking your knees, and so on. The fun will just be getting started when you realize that your hearts are pumping like mad and you're connecting with your kids in ways you never have before.

your family and friends, which can be very motivating and offer an added benefit—especially psychologically. Of course, giving yourself consistent recovery days is also part of a well-rounded workout routine, and in Chapters 9 and 10 we'll be going into the details of finding time to relax and settle your mind in ways that don't entail pumping your heart.

No matter which form or type of exercise you choose to do, its positive impact on your energy level—and looks and health—cannot be underestimated. Do you know any fit mother who doesn't look amazing and say she feels younger than she did ten years ago?

GETTING STARTED

Still don't know where to start? Are you sitting down reading this, terrified that you've cut your life short by staying on your butt all day long—yet the thought of exercise scares you?

If you're a true beginner, check out your local gym. Cardio classes are great if you need someone else to push you, and the energy of the other people in the class is sure to motivate you. Most gyms offer lots of choices, including step class, boot camps, indoor cycling, kickboxing, cardio dance class, and more. While you're there, check out the cardio equipment. But note: your body can adapt to these easily so the results you get in the first few months will no longer impress you. Keep changing it up. The recumbent bikes and the sit-up bikes are great for your legs and butt. The elliptical is awesome especially if you can crank the arms as well. Combining a workout with three different cardio machines is also a great way to kick up your heart rate as you know you will be moving on shortly. And if you're feeling intimidated, then have a trainer at your facility take you through a workout. Signing up for a short series of training sessions is not a bad idea as this will get you more familiar with the equipment and you'll feel more confident when it comes time for you to be on your own.

Here are a few more tips to make your move into working out regularly be as easy and effective as possible:

- **Pay attention to how you feel.** As you exercise, ask yourself: *Can I push harder? How am I breathing?* To have fun is to make your workouts a challenge.

- **Get meditative about it.** Find workouts that take you away. Listen to music that has a beat and rhythm to it that synchs with your workout. Create a playlist with songs that have a certain number of beats-per-minute depending on the type of workout you want to have. It's hard to pick up your pace if you're listening to Frank Sinatra.

- **Get a mentor or group of mentors.** Remember, group classes can help keep you stimulated and focused. Or get a friend who is in better shape than you and work out with her.

- **Hire a trainer.** We've said it before, but here it is again. A trainer can help keep you focused, busy, and motivated. You may need only one session to learn a comprehensive routine that you can repeat, modify, and improvise as you move forward.

- **Think whole body.** Visualize what your body parts do. Arms lift, push, pull, press, swing. So find machines that do those motions. Watch other people in the gym. Using the individual machines that focus on a particular body part is sometimes the best way to start. You want to hit arms, back, shoulders, chest, abs, legs (front and back), calves, and core.

- **Take a strength class.** A class where the instructor uses weights can help you learn positioning and how the exercise is supposed to feel as well as know what muscle you are working. This way when you get in the gym by yourself you will feel very comfortable picking up the free weights.

- **Try the kettlebells.** These are all the rage today but form and style are imperative to make this type of exercise effective. If your gym offers these classes, take one!

- **Go for new gadgets.** Gyms are typically filled with odd-looking gadgets—exercise balls, rubber tubing, ropes, jump ropes, foam rollers, etc.—that will add so much to your workouts. Before testing them out on your own, ask a trainer for help or check out the schedule for classes that teach you how to use them.

On a personal level, I feel better when the energy that I access in my work on a daily basis—i.e., my mind—is balanced by the energy that I access for exercise—my body. By balancing the two of them, I feel I can access the energy that nourishes my spirit.

After I became a mom, I needed exercise in so much more of a crucial way. Whereas I used to use exercise for the physical effects, I found that as a mother I looked to it for the mental benefits. Especially when you have three kids in the house at one time (!), it becomes difficult to feel like you're completing a task—let alone the 20 that you set out for yourself each day. I found that if I took an hour to walk the baby in the stroller and did a few sets of squats along the way, I felt a sense of accomplishment throughout the day that helped me battle postpartum blues and, later, just general mom-frustration!

— RACHEL LINCOLN SARNOFF,
executive director and CEO of Healthy Child Healthy World
and founder of www.EcoStiletto.com

Admit it: at some time or another, you've made the following declaration: "I'm so fat!" Maybe even in front of your kids without realizing it. It's hard to get away from the topic of weight in our society today. From endlessly hearing about the obesity epidemic to the latest trends in losing weight and hiding fat with fashion, the subject of weight just won't quit. It's pervasive and do we need to say it's also energy depleting? Hopefully this chapter has given you some ideas on ways in which you can rev your physical engine through exercise. But if the scientific benefits of exercise aren't enough to motivate you, then consider the other benefits: those that entail your commitment to your children and your positive self-image. Here's what we mean by that.

Obsessively thinking about weight seems to be par for the course these days among women. It's just too easy to slip into those thoughts even when we know deep down that they are not good for us, nor helpful. Consider the shallowness of that statement as you look at your child—your creation that was born from your amazing body. Every time the "I feel fat" statement zips through your brain, think of your beautiful children and learn to accept the body that has resulted. Granted, this doesn't imply that you cannot change your body and work toward having the body of your dreams. But don't let low-hanging comments like "I'm fat" derail your good intentions and psyche.

You have to look at the big picture—through your children's eyes or through your own ability—and rise above the lameness of statements like that. Instead, move in a direction of "I'm just going to do the best I can and be honest with what 'the best I can' means for me." How much will you let your muffin top really bother you? If you feel fabulous but cannot fit into size-2 jeans, isn't that okay? Having a skinny body isn't the goal—having a fully-functioning, vibrant body is.

Don't lose sight of your physical body. When you do there's a big disconnect from your neck down, and the types of problems that begin to present themselves at a very accelerated pace could be anything from knee problems to back problems to sleep issues, anxiety, overeating, boredom, and mood fluctuations. It's an over-used analogy, but looking at the body as a vehicle helps you to see why TLC is important. If you rely on your car to get you places, you are going to pay attention to its service. Similarly, the body is very resilient but there's only so much it can withstand without proper maintenance. And as you age, it will inevitably start to fall apart quicker.

There's energy in acceptance. Our youth-obsessed culture has us believing that younger is better. Giving in to that belief is draining. When you cannot accept who you are and where you are on your own spectrum of personal transformation, you cannot maximize your energy. And you cannot be the role model that your children deserve.

MOM UP! JUMP-START YOUR TRANSFORMATION

Getting into shape starts with just one mile. You can do this on a treadmill or take your GPS-equipped phone with you on a walk outside (or the old-fashioned method of mapping out a mile from your car's odometer so you know when to turn around). Alternatively, you can find a track at your local high school and walk around it four times. If you're on a treadmill, try putting your speed at 4.0 (four miles per hour) and see if you can keep up with that. If not, slow down. See how long it takes for you to do a full mile. Can you reach a mile in under 15 minutes? Make it a goal of just walking one mile at the start and then as you increase your speed, watch your time drop off. This is an indication that you're getting more fit. Ideally, a great walking workout is to walk three miles in fewer than 45 minutes. Don't hesitate to add intensity to your walks with handheld weights, hills (inclines and declines), stairs, and intervals of taking it up a notch and cranking hard for 10 minutes here and there.

CHAPTER 9

Refuel:
Bring Sleep into Your Night

Life as a mom is a shapeless blob of happy chaos.

— J U L I A   R O B E R T S

What your body does from the time it slips into bed to the time it wakes you up might have more to do with your energy metabolism than you realize. New findings in sleep medicine are currently revolutionizing how we think about the value sleep brings to our lives.

For so many moms we interviewed for this book, sleep ranked high on the list of priorities. Chaka Khan calls sleep "the key to a great energy balance"; Julia Roberts admits that any extra sleep she can get helps counterbalance the "mom struggle" that naturally accompanies having time thieves running around her house. Most of us just don't get the sleep we need. Sleep deprivation is epidemic. And let's face it: when we're sleep-deprived, moody, and things don't go our way, we can begin to go down that dreaded path that ends in depressive thoughts or a full-blown depression.

Moms in particular are starved for sleep, evidenced by the National Sleep Foundation's annual poll. The average woman aged 30 to 60 sleeps only six hours and 41 minutes per night during the workweek (less than the optimal eight to nine hours for health and wellness). On average, we get an hour less sleep per day than we did 40 years ago, and roughly two-thirds of us complain that sleep deprivation cuts into our life and well-being. In fact, sleep may have a greater influence on your ability to enjoy your day than household income and even marital status. One study found that an extra hour of sleep had more of an impact on how a group of women felt throughout the day than earning more money per year.

Without adequate sleep, not only does your entire body reel from its repercussions, but one system in particular—the endocrine, the center of gravity for a woman's energy levels—starts to malfunction. This can lead to everything from appetite and fat-storing hormones running amok to bona fide infertility.

Cutting-edge science now shows how critical sleep is to our ability to stay focused, learn new things and remember old things, lose fat and keep excess weight off, and generally lower the risks for a slew of health problems such as heart disease, obesity, and cerebrovascular disease. It also recharges us (duh!). But moms everywhere are burning the candle at both ends and leaving sleep last on their list. What's more, millions of moms struggle with chronic pain, high anxiety, or full-blown depression, and many become addicted to pain soothers such as alcohol or prescription pills, all of which further drain energy—including the energy required to get well.

Profile Alert! Wake up, Mom Zombie (Profile 2)! The information and ideas in this chapter should speak directly to you. Of course, we recommend that all the profile types heed this advice, but anyone who struggles to get a good night's sleep on a regular basis should really take this chapter to heart (and bed).

Today sleep medicine is a highly respected field of study that continues to provide alarming insights into the power of sleep in the support of health and energy. Sleep can dictate whether you can fight off infections, and how well you can cope with stress. We've already covered how sleep deprivation creates an imbalance of hormones that control your appetite and how your body burns energy. That's just the tip of the proverbial iceberg when it comes to associations between sleep and well-being.

Sleep is not a state of inactivity. It's not as if our bodies press pause for a few hours during the dark. Much to the contrary, a lot goes on during sleep at the cellular level to ensure that we can live another day. Clearly, a night of poor sleep or no sleep at all won't kill you, but prolonged sleep deprivation can have unintended consequences, not to mention putting you at high risk for an accident.

There's something to be said for looking refreshed and feeling smarter upon waking from a good night's sleep or a nap. Seemingly magical events happen when you're sleeping that just cannot happen during wakeful hours, and which help keep you energized and quick-witted. Proof of sleep's profound role in our lives also has been demonstrated over and over again in laboratory and clinical studies. It keeps you sharp, creative, and able to process information in an instant. Losing as few as one and a half hours for just one night reduces daytime alertness by about a third. And among the many side effects of poor sleep habits are hypertension, confusion, memory loss, the inability to learn new things, weight gain, obesity, cardiovascular disease, and depression.

One underappreciated aspect to sleep that is especially influential to our sense of well-being is its control of our hormonal cycles. Everyone has a biological, internal clock called a circadian rhythm (yes, even men can say they have a biological clock). It's the pattern of repeated activity associated with the environmental cycles of day and night—rhythms that repeat roughly every 24 hours. Examples include the sleep-wake cycle, the ebb and flow of hormones, the rise and fall of body temperature, and other subtle rhythms that mesh with the 24-hour solar day. When your rhythm is not in sync with the 24-hour solar day, you will feel (and probably look) it. Anyone who has traveled across time zones and felt off-kilter for a few days can understand this.

So much of our circadian rhythm revolves around our sleep habits. A healthy day-night cycle is tied into our normal hormonal secretion patterns, from those associated with our eating patterns to those that relate to stress and cellular recovery. Cortisol, for example, should be highest in the morning and progressively decrease throughout the day, with the lowest levels occurring after 11 P.M. With (hopefully) low evening cortisol levels, melatonin levels rise. This is the hormone that tells you it's time to sleep; it helps regulate your 24-hour circadian rhythm, alerting your brain that it's dark outside. Once released, it slows body function, lowers blood pressure, and, in turn, core body temperature so you're prepared to sleep. Higher melatonin levels will allow for more deep sleep, which helps maintain healthy levels of growth hormone, thyroid hormone, and sex hormones. All good things for keeping up appearances and energy levels.

> If you've ever had a tough time winding down at night due to stress, you may be secreting too much cortisol, which competes with the sleep-enhancing melatonin.

Why You Need to Go Deep

Lots of hormones are associated with sleep, some of which rely on sleep to get released. As soon as you hit deep sleep, about 20 to 30 minutes after you first close your eyes, and then a couple more times throughout the night in your sleep cycle, your pituitary gland at the base of your brain releases high levels of growth hormone (GH)—the most it's going to secrete in 24 hours.

Growth hormone does more than just stimulate growth and cell reproduction; it also refreshes cells, restores skin's elasticity, and enhances the movement of amino acids through cell membranes. Growth hormone aids in your ability to maintain an ideal weight, too, effectively telling your cells to back off on using carbs for energy and use fat instead. Without adequate sleep, GH stays locked up in the pituitary, which negatively affects your proportions of fat to muscle. Over time, low GH levels are associated with high fat and low lean muscle.

Growth hormone affects almost every cell in the body, renewing the skin and bones; regenerating the heart, liver, lungs, and kidneys; and bringing back organ and tissue function to more youthful levels. Growth hormone also revitalizes the immune system, lowers the risk factors of heart attack and stroke, improves oxygen uptake, and even helps prevent osteoporosis.

> **Sleep on this:** The trouble with running up sleep shortages day after day is that it's very hard to make up the loss unless you're going on vacation. What's more, when sleep is skimpy, your cortisol levels don't drop as much as they're supposed to at night, and growth hormone doesn't rise as much as it should, which can undermine muscle strength. Remember, you need a daily dose of growth hormone, which gets secreted during deep sleep, to refresh your cells and prepare you for the next day. It not only stimulates cellular growth and reproduction, but it also has strong anti-inflammatory, antifat, and anticortisol effects—all good things for energy (not to mention weight maintenance!).

How Does Sleep Happen?

It's one of those fundamental questions that have plagued scientists for a very long time. As we were writing this book yet another study emerged to help explain how the body knows to flip the switch and go from wakefulness to a sleep state. It turns out that those fundamental molecules of energy that literally charge our cells—ATP—take center stage. Washington State University researchers documented how active brain cells release ATP to start the events leading to sleep. The ATP then binds to a receptor responsible for cell processing and the release of cytokines, small signaling proteins involved in sleep regulation. By charting the link between ATP and the sleep-regulatory substances, the researchers found the way in which the brain keeps track of activity and ultimately switches from a wakeful to sleeping state. For example, learning and memory depend on changing the connections between brain cells. The study shows that ATP is the signal behind those changes. Pretty cool stuff, and once again a reminder that energy has as much to do with how we feel during our waking minutes as it does with how well we sleep at night and prepare for another active day.

THE MAGIC NUMBER

It's a myth that there's a magic number of hours the body requires to sleep. Everyone has a different sleep need. The eight-hour rule is general, but not necessarily the ideal number for you. Most people need seven to nine hours, and chances are you know what your number is. If you feel like a drag after a six-hour night, then clearly you need to aim for more sleep. Think of the last time you went on vacation and slept like a baby for more hours a night than usual. That is probably your perfect number. Poor sleep catches up to most of us, and it's practically impossible to make up a sleep loss because life keeps moving forward and demanding more of us. Despite what many people attempt to do, shifting your sleep habits on the weekends to catch up can sabotage a healthy circadian rhythm.

Not surprisingly, stress and staying up too late are the two big culprits to poor sleep, which is why it's important to establish what's called a healthy "sleep hygiene"—the habits that make for a restful night's sleep regardless of factors such as age and underlying medical conditions that can disrupt sleep. The goal is to minimize those factors' effects on us so we can welcome peaceful sleep.

12 PATHS TO PERFECT SLEEP

1. **Get on a schedule.** Go to bed and wake up at the same time seven days a week, weekends included. Try not to fall into a cycle of burning the midnight oil on Sunday night in preparation for Monday, letting your sleep debt pile up for the week and then attempt to catch up on sleep over the weekend. It won't work. Stick to the same schedule seven days a week. Your body and energy levels will love it.

2. **Unplug to recharge.** Set aside at least 30 minutes before bedtime to unwind and prepare for sleep. Avoid stimulating activities (e.g., work, cleaning, being on the computer, watching TV dramas that get your adrenaline running). Try soaking in a warm bath or engaging in some light stretching. Once you're in bed, do some light reading and push any anxieties aside.

3. **Don't let your To Do list or worries take control.** Early in the evening—say, right after dinner—write out tasks you have yet to complete that week (not tonight!) and prioritize them realistically. Add any particular worries you might have. If these notes begin to talk to you when you're trying to go to sleep, tell yourself it's time to focus on sleep. Everything will be okay. You're tired and will have a productive day tomorrow. You're relaxed and at peace. The body needs to sleep and is ready for it.

4. **Create a restful refuge.** Reserve the bedroom for sleep (and sex) only. Remove distracting electronics and gadgets and keep it clean, cool, and dark.

5. **Nix the fix and cut the caffeine.** Stop drinking caffeinated beverages about eight hours before bedtime. Due to caffeine's half-life (how long it takes for caffeine to lose half of its punch in your body), you'll need all that time to let your body process all the caffeine so it won't infringe upon restful sleep. If you cannot go cold turkey on the caffeine in the afternoon, then switch to drinks with less caffeine, such as teas.

6. **Don't sweat it.** Watch out if you exercise within three hours of bedtime. For some people, exercise can be stimulating to the point it affects getting to bed on time and falling asleep easily. This is when tracking your sleep experiences and what you do beforehand can help you to pinpoint your own unique culprits to restless sleep. If your body's reaction to exercise is stealing your sleep, then shift your exercise to earlier in the day.

7. **Limit your libations.** Be cautious about alcohol intake in the evening hours. If you use a glass of wine as a way to unwind after the kids have gone to bed, which is how many moms decompress at the end of the day, be mindful of how that glass (or two) could be influencing the quality of your sleep. You might want to test out avoiding this routine and see if it changes how refreshed you feel the next day.

8. **Ditch digestive distractions.** Keep in mind that heavy foods too close to bedtime can upset your sleep as much as they upset your stomach. The best bedtime snack is nothing. Eating provides energy and that runs counter to prepping the body for rest. If you

need to take a medication or if you are breastfeeding and up during the night, then maybe a liquid such as plain coconut water will satisfy you. This requires no extra digestive work; it's a diluted amount of carbohydrates that also provides potassium for hydration, which will help the body with recovery. To balance it out, you could have 10 to 15 nuts with it.

9. **Focus on relaxing.** Try valerian herbal tea or a chamomile blend before bedtime. Take your magnesium supplement in the evening hours to help relax muscles for better sleep and regularity.

10. **Practice aromatherapy.** Keep a sachet of lavender by your bed and take a whiff before hitting the pillow. Lavender has known sleep-inducing effects. Other aromas widely considered to be relaxing are rose, vanilla, and lemongrass—but different ones work for different people. For you, maybe lavender is stimulating and rose is not. Scented lotions can also be effective.

11. **Take a d-e-e-p breath . . . and release.** On your back with your eyes closed and your body stretched out, hands by your sides, palms facing up, begin to squeeze and release your muscles, starting with your head and face and working down to your toes. Breathe in deeply and slowly, telling yourself, *I will fall asleep. I am going to sleep.*

12. **Get out of the bedroom.** We all think that if we lie in bed long enough, sleep will come. Instead, our minds tend to get busier and our muscles tenser as we stress over being awake. Give it a rest. If you can't get to sleep within 20 minutes, slip out of bed and go to a safe haven—a place that's comfy, has dim lighting, and no distractions. Just sit comfortably.

Or do your breathing exercises. Or read. No e-mail, TV, or other electronics though. The point is to give your mind-body a respite from trying so hard to nod off. After 20 minutes or so, go back to bed and see what happens when you're more relaxed. Repeat once or twice if necessary.

Do sleep aids aid? There are plenty of pill pushers these days in the sleep department. From over-the-counter remedies to prescriptions marketed as nonaddictive and safe, sleep aids are a gigantic industry. Choosing to go that route is totally up to you, but be aware of the potential downsides, including those related to energy metabolism. Modern sleep medications are not all they are cracked up to be. They may not be as chemically addicting as earlier generations of sleep drugs, but they can be psychologically addicting. What's more, they can prevent you from reaching the furthest reaches of deep sleep for long enough to reap all of its rewards. They may also make you groggy or feel hungover the next day.

You'll be amazed by the power of sleep when it comes naturally just by regulating your sleep habits. You body will respond and adapt to the sleep cycle you put it on. If your body clock is truly off, try getting some natural morning sunlight on you, do some exercise during the day, don't stay up until the wee hours of the morning cleaning house, and set aside time to wind down before bedtime. Yes, it's as simple as that!

Got Too Much Negative Energy?

One more note before moving on: sometimes our sleep troubles are hiding more profound problems which surface late at night, stirring insomnia. Let's call it negative energy, and this can entail any number of loaded guns—body-image issues, feeling inadequate as a mother or wife, health concerns, failures in your relationships, disappointments at work, worries about money and financial strife, struggles with juggling your parents' health and raising your own children, etc. Go ahead and think of what keeps you up at night. We all have our lists. And they can be long.

Don't think for a minute that these matters don't play into our energy equation. They will pull down any bit of good energy and sabotage it into a very dark and negative place. They can bleed into every part of your being—your relationships with your kids, spouse, friends, job, yourself. Letting these dilemmas simmer in our minds is so worthless, and it gets us nowhere. It also eventually leads us to degrade ourselves. And our bodies hear it, immediately downshifting to preserve precious energy.

In the next and final chapter, we'll delve into the secrets to managing stress, which will play into your ability to get a good night's rest. When you do find yourself churning awful thoughts, turn it around and say something positive about yourself and your commitment to make positive change. For every negative thing you say about yourself and any "predicament" you might find yourself in, say three positive things. I hate my legs. I love my elbows. I love my chin. I love my hair. I hate my job. I love my children. I love my courage. I love my strength. Self-esteem and self-confidence are very powerful. They are also very energizing.

MOM UP! JUMP-START YOUR TRANSFORMATION

Of all the ideas we've given to help you get a good night's sleep, one of the most essential (and least followed) is the one about setting aside time to wind down before bedtime. Far too often, moms find themselves doing last-minute chores and tasks long after the day should have been declared over. Once the kids go to bed, don't give yourself permission to use the rest of the night to catch up on everything else at the expense of a full night's sleep. So if you want just one thing to do differently, see if you can—for one week, hopefully longer—allocate *one hour* before your bedtime during which you don't engage in any stimulating activities such as e-mail, Internet surfing, or even watching television. Instead, opt for a hot soak in your bathtub, reading, or spending time with your spouse. If one hour is unrealistic, then try it for a few days and then cut it back to 30 minutes. But no less! This is You Time, and you'll notice a difference in the quality of your sleep.

CHAPTER 10

Have Fun:
Learn the Power of Play

I feel there are two people inside me—me and my intuition.
If I go against her, she'll screw me every time, and if I follow her,
we get along quite nicely.

— K I M   B A S I N G E R

Kim Basinger is by far the one who adheres to the utmost perfect nutrition and a regular exercise routine no matter what's going on in her life. She lives with pure dedication. No sidetracks. It's a mind-set for her that never wavers. "You decide this is the way I'm going to live my life and you stick with it," she says. "You live it, you breathe it, and you do it."

Not everyone can adhere to Kim's stoic way of living, but she affords us a role model by which to compare values and priorities. Too many women let motherhood prevent them from taking care of themselves. In this final chapter we drive home the power of play—giving yourself regular permission to put yourself first and routinely pamper yourself. Only then can you recharge maximally and amplify your capacity to fulfill that role as Mommy. After all, the body needs playtime. It's what nature intended.

Playtime is what ultimately allows us to manage our biggest, and most wily, adversary in our pursuit of more energy: stress. We could have easily based the whole book around the effects stress can have on our energy, but decided to save this topic for last. By now, you've already gained a tremendous amount of information about the body's chemistry and energy metabolism. We hope you've already turned the volume down on your stress level just by incorporating some of our strategies. But we need to expand on stress's far-reaching implications that can do way more than just sap your energy from a superficial standpoint. For some of you, this chapter's ideas could very well be your starting point for change. Why? Because the secret to getting more energy could very well begin with simply admitting that you don't have any energy, for which starting with recovery (ahem: relaxation) first is required. Alcoholics who participate in the classic 12-step program have to admit the problem, which is their first baby step to a sober life. So it's something to consider: achieving an energetic life might start just with taking the sting out of your stress.

> **Profile Alert!** The Overscheduled and the Dead Battery will want to read this chapter twice. That's right: if you're Profile 3 or 5, chances are you never find a spare moment to play. And it's about time that you did.

A COMMON DENOMINATOR TO LACK OF ENERGY

Stress's impact on all things physiological, mental, psychological, and spiritual are well documented. And remarkable. Innumerable studies have shown a direct link between stress and weight gain, for instance; stress can drain your energy simply by taxing your metabolism and flooding the body with stress hormones that weaken your whole energy equation. In studies, more than 70 percent of those who undereat or overeat during a stressful period admit to snacking on foods that are nutrient poor. Fats and sugars seem to fit the bill during times of stress.

New research from Germany shows that people who had heart attacks were three times more likely than not to have been sitting in traffic an hour before their symptoms began. And for some strange reason not identified yet, a woman's risk of heart attack is five times higher within an hour of being in traffic.

This scenario, coupled with our society's increasing financial troubles, has a far-reaching domino effect. To make more money to pay for living expenses, we are working longer hours. Stay-at-home moms don't get a free pass, either. In fact, the mother who devotes all of her time to caring for the needs of her children may be shouldering more stress than the mom who can escape to an office. Unfortunately, stay-at-home moms often don't feel they have the right to be stressed, or that somehow their stress isn't validated so therefore doesn't count.

Suffice it to say, whether you're a working mother or not, we are accepting an unprecedented level of stress in our lives. All of this has put a great strain on our health and well-being, especially because the vast majority of Americans are barely keeping up. So it's not surprising that over the past few years doctors in all fields of medicine have seen a dramatic change in their patients' stress levels. Stress is at the top of the metaphorical food chain—tripping a cascade of events that can lead to thicker waistlines, dour moods, poor sleep, chronic inflammation, and oxidative stress, and, as a result, an unhealthy body and energy level.

On the positive side, if stress is such an influential cast member in our world, and we can learn how to control it with the help of our lifestyle choices, then we may be able to champion the balancing act so we achieve peak health and energy. And that's exactly what we're going to do. Let's take a quick tour of your body's stress-response system and then see how we can lighten the load.

> Stress is an issue, but *the* issue is our inability to relax—to learn to turn *off* the stress.

THE SCIENCE OF STRESS

From an evolutionary and survivalist perspective, stress is a good thing. It's supposed to prime the body for battle and get us out of harm's way. The problem, though, is that our physical reaction is the same every time we sense a potential threat, whether it's real and coming from something truly life-threatening, or just the To Do list and screaming kids.

First, the brain signals to the adrenal glands to release epinephrine, better known as adrenaline. This is what causes your heart to pick up speed as blood rushes to your muscles in case you need to make a run for it. That adrenaline, by the way, steals blood from the skin and face to allocate it toward your muscles, which is why you can suddenly look pale as a ghost or become white with fear.

As soon as the threat passes, your body returns to normal. If the threat doesn't pass and your stress response gets stronger, then a whole wave of stress hormones gets released in a series of events along the hypothalamic-pituitary-adrenal (HPA) axis. The hypothalamus, a region of the brain, first releases a stress coordinator called corticotropin-releasing hormone (CRH). The hypothalamus is frequently referred to as the seat of our emotions. It's our chief leader in emotional processing. The split second you feel anxious, deeply worried, scared, or simply concerned that you can't pay a bill, the hypothalamus secretes CRH to start a domino effect ending in cortisol rushing into your bloodstream.

We've already mentioned cortisol—it's the body's chief stress hormone, aiding in that famous fight-or-flight response. It also controls how your body processes carbs, fats, and proteins, and helps it to reduce inflammation. Because it's the hormone responsible for protecting you, its actions increase your appetite, tell your body to stock up on more fat, and break down materials that can be used for quick forms of energy, including muscle. Not all that you'd like to happen, but when your body senses stress (even when you know it's not the kind that will physically kill you in ten seconds or less), it thinks you won't see food again for a while—or it may need an ample supply of fuel to camp out on during a famine or use to make a mad dash. In other words, cortisol causes tissues to break down, including muscle, skin, and collagen, while at the same time assembling fat.

For this reason, excessive cortisol levels can wreak havoc on the body, making it hard to lose weight, replenish cells, encourage the growth of new cells, and form new youth-building collagen. Excess cortisol over time can lead to increased abdominal fat, irritability and full-blown depression, bone loss, a suppressed immune system, fatigue, and an increased risk for insulin resistance, diabetes, and heart disease just to name a few things. Everything takes a hit, including blood vessels that become more fragile and can't keep meeting demands. Cortisol does, however, serve a positive role. It helps immune cells attack infectious invaders and tells the brain when those invaders have been taken care of. And another way to look at its effects in mobilizing fat and upping your appetite is that it builds up energy reserves (calories) that your muscles may need soon. But for the most part, you don't need those energy reserves because you're not in dire straits. You're just overreacting to a trivial stressor that your body interprets as something serious. But it has a profound impact on you regardless.

The scientific study of the impact of stress on the body from the inside out, and even the outside in, has made tremendous advances in the past decade. In 1998, doctors from Harvard University conducted a joint study with several Boston-area hospitals designed to examine the connections and interactions between the mind and the body, specifically the skin. They dubbed their findings the NICE network, which stands for neuro-immuno-cutaneous-endocrine. In plain speak, it's a network consisting of your nervous system, immune system, skin, and endocrine (hormonal) system. All of these are intimately connected through a dialogue of shared interactive chemicals. Like a giant wireless network, when one phone rings, the others can hear it and respond.

The Boston researchers studied how various external forces affect our state of mind, from massage and aromatherapy to depression and isolation. What they discovered confirmed what we had already known anecdotally for centuries: our state of mind has a definite impact on our health and even our looks. People suffering from depression, for example, look older and less healthy, and not because they've let themselves go and aren't grooming themselves as rigorously as their happier counterparts. But they actually are older than happier comrades who are the same biological age. The stress of living with depression has accelerated the aging process and damaged their health.

Depression is not something to take lightly. One of the more troubling pieces of news to come out recently is the fact that depression will have a huge impact on our world in the future. The World Health Organization has estimated that by the year 2020, depression will be the second leading disability-causing disease in the world. In many developed countries, such as the United States, depression is already among the top causes in terms of disability and excess mortality.

Take time for yourself. Don't let yourself go. Exercise, eat well, and get a manicure or pedicure once in a while. Stay connected to what is important to you. Make time for your marriage or with your partner, make time for each other without discussing work or your kids—it's a chance to grow closer.

Being a mother never ends. It's a gift that we are given to learn about who we are and how we show up in the world.

— **MARIEL HEMINGWAY,**
mother of two, author, yogi, and spokesperson for green living

---

Ways to Relax and Rev Energy

You already know in your heart that taking care of yourself sets the tone of your life and health. It sounds almost cliché to say you need to relax because it will reduce stress, since this is like telling someone not to breathe (or check e-mail). Stress will always be a part of our life—and our livelihood. The key is to keep certain sources of unnecessary stress at bay so they don't affect us like a charging rhino. Easier said than done, but here are some strategies to consider.

Be brutal about boundaries. We talked a lot about boundaries throughout this book, but how well have you been able to live up to our recommendations? Can you set a time each day after which you turn off your electronics and don't respond to nonemergency calls, e-mails, text messages, and so on? Can you create a bedtime routine that prepares you for sleep 30 to 60 minutes prior to lights out? Can you plan your days better so you're not as harried? When you create (and stick to) boundaries that help you to achieve better health, you'll increase your chances at optimizing your energy. You can make boundaries for yourself in all areas of your life, from what time you choose to get up (or, on the other side of the day, go to bed) to what you buy in the supermarket and how many days you'll let go by without exercising.

Find your inner scribe. Okay, so maybe you're not a writer, a blogger, or someone who keeps a journal. We're not asking you to be any of those, but you'd be surprised by what taking just three to five minutes at the end or start of your day can do. Use it to evaluate how you feel and what you're thinking at a subconscious level and watch what it does to your sense of well-being, peace of mind, and even your capacity to dream big, set realistic goals for the future, and realize optimal energy. So few of us take the time anymore during our days serving and caring for others to turn the volume down on everyone and everything else and just think in our own creative space and quietude.

Self-care begins with self-discovery. And committing your thoughts and ideas to paper can make a huge difference. It affords you a record from which to look back in the future and simultaneously offers accountability. It also gives you a chance to adjust your attitudes if need be and set a new course that moves you closer to where you want to be. Find a comfortable spot (or just do this exercise while sitting in bed) and consider playing some relaxing music.

You may find it helpful to keep more than one journal. Have one that you use to write down the more mundane tasks you need to get done, such as picking up clothes from the cleaners, grocery shopping, or organizing a birthday party. Have another that keeps track of your diet choices and physical activities. Yet another journal, a so-called worry journal, can be very handy for people who have a hard time getting to sleep at night as stressful thoughts intrude and steal much-needed sleep time. A worry journal by your bedside can act as a mental depository of your anxieties. Once you write them down, you close the book and tell yourself that you will deal with them tomorrow. Sometimes you'll find that the act of writing down a worry will lead to solutions that you never thought of before. And all of these exercises will subconsciously give you hope for your future.

Last but certainly not least, keep a positive-note journal that tracks all the good things you've accomplished. At the end of even the most stressful days, stop to reflect on what went right. What are you grateful for? What good things came out of the day, even if they were unplanned or unexpected? Sometimes, on the worst of days, we can just be thankful that we got through it, and soon we can embrace a whole new day with happy, promising thoughts and intentions.

Sounds ridiculous, but take a walk. I always found that getting outside my house when I was in almost any mood made for more energy and creativity. Even if it was around the block. Studies prove it, but anecdotally it is true. It is also hard to be sad or unhappy when strolling outside in nature. All the while the residual effects strengthen bones, burn calories, and boost feelings of happiness, so walk on! In addition—have a snack in your purse. My body tends to need fuel every two hours, so I found keeping a small snack with me helps energy levels stay even, which in turn kept me from unnecessarily yelling at my child.

— LORI CORBIN

ABC7 Los Angeles' Food and Fitness Coach,
and host of Live Well HD's *Custom Fit*

Try something new. Remember how exciting that first day of school was back when you were entering the third or fourth grade? It's thrilling to enter a new environment, meet new people, and learn something different. Women trying to keep up with their everyday obligations rarely give themselves permission to act like schoolgirls again, but doing so can have some surprising benefits. In addition to expanding your horizons and exposing yourself to a new hobby or skill, trying something new can take you just far enough away from your established and routine commitments to give you the feeling that you're on vacation, that you're allowed to goof off and replenish the kid in you again that's unencumbered by the banalities of everyday life.

Think about your current hobbies or one you'd like to try, and see if you can find a club, group, or class nearby in which to participate. This can be any number of things, including cooking class, a writing class, a pottery workshop, a photo club, a class for learning a new language, or a book club. And if you can't find anything attuned to your interests, then start your own club or group and invite your friends.

Trying something new can also mean seeking a new setting. Go for a walk and call a friend you haven't spoken with in a long while, get on a bicycle, take an exercise class, jump rope for a solid minute or get 100 revolutions without missing, make a pot of green tea and then sit by a window and flip through a magazine, take a cat nap in the sun. Do something that gets you out of your normal routine.

Take (a few) deep breaths. Deep breathing techniques can yank you out of a blue mood quickly. Slow, controlled breathing is the foundation for many Eastern practices such as yoga, qigong, tai chi, and classic meditation—all of which aim to plunge the body (and mind, clearly) into a balanced, stress-free state. One of the reasons why deep breathing is so helpful is that it triggers a parasympathetic nerve response, as opposed to a sympathetic nerve response, the latter of which is sensitive to stress and anxiety. At the onset of stress, the sympathetic nervous system springs into action and is largely responsible for those oft-damaging spikes in the stress hormones cortisol and adrenaline. The parasympathetic nervous system, on the other hand, can trigger a relaxation response, and deep breathing is the quickest means of getting these two systems to communicate. You can flip the switch from high alert to low in seconds as your heart rate slows, muscles relax, and blood pressure lowers.

Meditation, which entails deep breathing, also has mind-altering benefits. The practice casts the human brain back to its pre-neocortex state, allowing us to be freed of our analytical selves. In this blissful state, one is aware of senses, feelings, and state of mind—without the negativity. We lead very scatterbrained lives, wrapped up in the frenzied competition that is our society—and momhood. We rarely take the time to sit and concentrate on ourselves without the dramas of being a mother affecting us. No wonder meditation is so effective just by virtue of its permission to let us be mindful, centered, and focused. It appears that meditation is truly exercise for the brain, as if it helps grow stronger "muscles" in the areas used.

The Breath of Fire. Can you take a recess for some deep breathing or meditation when problems present themselves and your mind starts to race? Problems can easily swell into unmanageable portion sizes for our consciousness and bring us down. Then they get out of control and look worse than they really are. Deep breathing or meditation will help you to gain perspective and reclaim sanity again. The following exercise is adapted from a yogic breathing technique. Its aim is to raise vital energy and increase alertness, and can be done anytime you need to feel rejuvenated in less than 60 seconds.

1. Inhale and exhale rapidly through your nose, keeping your mouth closed but relaxed. Your breaths in and out should be equal in duration, but as short as possible. This is a noisy breathing exercise.

2. Do not do for more than 15 seconds on your first try. Each time you practice the Breath of Fire, you can increase your time by 5 seconds or so, until you reach a full minute.

3. If done properly, you will feel invigorated, comparable to the heightened awareness you feel after a good workout. You should feel the effort at the back of the neck, the diaphragm, the chest, and the abdomen. Try this breathing exercise the next time you need an energy boost and feel yourself reaching for a cup of coffee.

Recent studies have shown that yoga and meditation, practiced for three months, reduced waist circumference, systolic blood pressure, and fasting blood sugar and triglyceride levels. It also increased levels of high-density lipoprotein (the good fats). In addition, at the end of the study periods, feelings of anxiety, stress, and depression were significantly decreased, and optimism was significantly increased. That all spells more energy. The researchers concluded that yoga not only helps in prevention of lifestyle diseases, but can also be a powerful adjunct therapy when diseases occur.

Deep breathing can be done anywhere, anytime. Sit comfortably in a chair or lie down.

Close your eyes and make sure your body is relaxed, releasing all tension in your neck, arms, legs, and back. Inhale through your nose for as long as you can, feeling your diaphragm and abdomen rise as your stomach moves outward. Sip in a little more air when you think you've reached the top of your lungs. Slowly exhale to a count of 20, pushing every breath of air from your lungs. Continue for at least five rounds of deep breaths.

Plan your personal days, even if it's just for ten minutes. When you map out your week in advance, figure out when you'll be able to set aside time for just you—no kids, no demands, no work. Be brutal with your time and make it happen no matter what. You never know, you just might find a full extra hour to treat yourself to a massage or another therapeutic treatment of your choice. When you plan, extra time finds you. Use it for just you.

Remember, we're people with lives independent from our kids, and we need to put ourselves first on a regular basis so we can enjoy (and not resent) the wonderful families we are lucky enough to be a part of. A day of golf, lunch and a movie with friends, a weekend trip to visit a college buddy—whatever! You have to trust that the world goes on without you and it's okay for your husband and kids to cover for you.

Grab the great outdoors. Enjoy the calming effects that only nature can provide. So few of us spend time outdoors anymore. We live and work indoors, often chained to electronics, meetings, and chores. But being outdoors and among plants and other living things can enhance feelings of health and well-being. This is partly why going for walks and hikes, or sailing, skiing, cycling—doing anything in the open air—can be so invigorating. Don't forget to bring the outdoors in, too. Park a big, live plant in the room where you spend the most time each day (philodendrons are nearly impossible to kill). Set up a reading chair beside a window where you can observe trees and birds.

Soak in a dose of morning light. Our body clocks don't exactly match the day's 24-hour-day clock, which makes us want to sleep about 12 minutes longer every day and stay up later every night. What helps? Getting out of bed at the same time every morning and sitting in a sunny spot for breakfast, or exercising outdoors, or just turning on lots of lights. A dose of brightness in the morning helps synch up your internal clock with the 24-hour day. Which also helps you get on a regular, saner schedule.

Ask for help. Trade babysitting nights with family or friends. Ask your spouse to pick up more slack. Single moms need to be even more vigilant with their time and energy, and not hesitate to call on friends and family for help. Nearly half of working mothers are heavily stressed every day. It takes a village to raise children, but many parents are doing it solo. Do what you need to do in order to have more *you* time.

By the same token, don't play "helicopter" parent. Start your children at an early age performing age-related tasks that make life easier. Get them to make their own breakfast, clean their rooms, and place their things in proper spots. Less chaos is helpful for everyone. Shower them with love, but send them to bed on their own after second grade. The bedtime situation is usually challenging.

Be attentive to the state of your health at all times.
Paying attention to my self-care informs everything I do.
If I'm not taking care of myself, how can I take care of others?
And by taking care of yourself you set an example for your
children on how important self-care is.

— S H E L P I N K ,

mother and founder of SpaRitual

Share the vibe. Schedule a dinner club once a month with your friends—people with whom you share deep connections. Setting aside time with those who can help us relax and move away from the limelight of stress is important for our emotional and physical health. As we mentioned earlier, it's important for us as women to get together and talk, share stories and advice, and laugh. It's a great way to decompress. Once a month, plan your outings with your friends (where, when, who is hosting, who is cooking, etc.) and don't let a month go by without one of these get-togethers. Maybe you'll just sit around playing Bunko or listening to music and drinking wine. However the night plays itself out, you'll come to enjoy these times together—and so will your body's energy-making machine. Warning: talking on the phone doesn't count here. Even though we have more gadgets now than ever to connect with others, we also have a higher number of people complaining of loneliness and feelings of disconnectedness. It seems like the more connections we make on the surface, the more we lose out on opportunities to nourish and renew those much deeper and rewarding connections in person.

Be your own cheerleader. Before you have to take care of anyone else in your day, take care of you first by giving yourself a morning pep talk while you're in front of the mirror. It may seem silly, but saying a few positive affirmations, such as "I'm going to have a fabulous day; I'm full of untapped energy and health, and it's up to me to make great things happen" has hidden benefits. Even if you don't quite believe yourself, it's still effective. Research has shown that over time, a daily rah-rah builds resilience, which can fortify you against stress.

Laugh more. Even if you have to force yourself to laugh, it's worth it. The health benefits of laughter are proven and plentiful, ranging from strengthening the immune system to reducing stress and food cravings to increasing one's threshold for pain. Hormones, of course, are the reason. Health-promoting endorphins and neurotransmitters get released during a good laugh, and the number of antibody-producing cells and the effectiveness of certain immune cells also increase. An emerging therapeutic field known as humor therapy aims to help people heal more quickly with laughter.

Give back. Have you ever signed up to volunteer in community events? Have you ever offered your time and expertise to a local youth club or adult-education center? Have you ever joined a mentorship program that matches you with another individual who wants to learn your skills? Have you ever watched a group of volunteers cleaning up a park or beach and wished you could join them? There are dozens of ways you can give back. Though the media likes to focus on how giving back is the practical way in which each one of us can have an impact in the world and effect global change, think about what it gives the person who is doing the giving back: a chance to forge new friendships, to squelch feelings of isolation and stress, and to enjoy the act of making a difference that will surely make a difference on a much smaller—yes, energetic—level.

Don't have time to volunteer? Then try this: adopt a sister from around the world through an organization such as Women for Women International.

Get out of your world. Maybe it's planting succulents in funky pots or shopping for vintage clothing. If you're like one of us, perhaps it's buying *Country Living* magazine to find ideas for rearranging furniture and creating new sitting areas in your home. Find a crafty, silly activity that takes you out of your world. Make it a ritual as often as you can. Denise Richards loves to volunteer at animal shelters. For her, it's a relaxing diversion and removes her from the rigors of daily life. Best of all, it doesn't require any money and involves physical work. And that's key. See if you can find a hobby that pushes you a little past your comfort zone, engages your creativity, costs little or nothing, and challenges you to try something different for a change. It could be as simple as flipping through a stack of favorite photographs. Can't think of anything? Then just try this: after the kids have gone to bed, fill the bathtub, light candles, and slowly sip a cup of hot tea or glass of wine as you read a book for an hour. See how that makes you feel. Experiment with activities that cleanse your mood, from aromatherapy to visualization.

Dare to disconnect. There's a strange duality to being attached to machines that allow us to connect with others around the world in an instant. From cell phones to social networks that can transmit what you're doing right now in fractions of a second, communication these days is quick, easy, and, to a large degree, isolating. When you resort to electronic transmissions of information rather than speaking to someone in person or even over the phone, you lose a human touch to the experience. You also have a tendency to lose focus, as those transmissions become rapid-fire, frequent, distracting, and intrusive. We admire people who make a choice to carve out time once or twice a week when they put down their smartphones and don't check their e-mail. It can be incredibly invigorating and stress-reducing to disconnect yourself occasionally from the digital world. See if you can designate a single day a week, perhaps a whole weekend from time to time, when you let the voice mail and the e-mail pile up. Detach yourself from the need to keep checking and responding to the constant, chattering influx—much of which is not important, not urgent, and not helpful to your health and well-being.

You can always find 30 to 60 seconds. Thirty to 60 seconds of deep breathing while concentrating on following your breath is a quick but very restorative meditation. Same for a short stretch. And if you can take 15 minutes for a power nap, the world looks different. Hug your kids, husband, and friends a lot. And pay 100 percent attention when you do. At the end of the day, write a list of anything you need to get done in the near future that weighs on your mind, put it aside, and then think of all you enjoyed and accomplished that day. Gratitude is a great antidote to frustration and upset.

— MYRA GOODMAN,

co-founder of Earthbound Farm,
cookbook author, and mom

Move more. The power of exercise in reducing stress is well known. But here's something you might not have known: exercise makes your blood circulate more quickly, transporting the stress hormone (and fat-friendly) cortisol to your kidneys and flushing it out of your system. Remember, cortisol encourages your body to store fat—especially visceral fat—that releases fatty acids into your blood, raising cholesterol and insulin levels and paving the way for heart disease and diabetes. One study found that 18 minutes of walking three times per week can quickly lower the hormone's levels by 15 percent!

Be still. For most of us, life is so scheduled, speedy, and "on" that we never do absolutely nothing. It's rare to set aside time to simply be—no agenda, no demands, no plan. So find a comfortable, quiet spot to sit for five to ten minutes every day, stop all your hustling and bustling . . . and simply, by yourself, be still. Slowing down in this way, if you do it every day, helps create a sense of spaciousness in your life, a break in the old routine. It can open the door to new perceptions, new solutions to old problems, and new possibilities. It gives your brain, your psyche, your whole being a break. Like one long peaceful sigh.

Bust a bad day. Having a really bad day? End it! Sometimes we can't fix a day that's gone really bad. The sooner you can end it, the sooner you can leave it behind and start afresh again. And if it's too early to end it, then try a nap to reboot yourself—and your day. Be careful how your bad day is affecting your decisions (e.g., what you eat, how you behave in front of your children, and so on). Don't trade one bandage for another, such as soothing your bad day with an outrageous shopping spree that sinks your bank account. Continue to make informed decisions that feed your energy tank so you don't feel like a victim but you also don't feel deprived. Don't be afraid to cry! If you feel like it, it's a great option.

Sex it up. Who doesn't feel more energized after a night of great sex? If sex didn't do a body good, then it wouldn't make us feel so fantastic and crave the next session. That's right: for once, something that feels good is actually good for us. Sex makes us happy, and great sex in a loving, intimate relationship makes us even happier. For starters, sex is one of the world's best stress releasers, and as with almost everything else that we've been talking about, it all comes down to hormones—those chemical messengers that dictate how we feel. Beta-endorphins, prolactin, and oxytocin wash through you during sex. Beta-endorphin is a natural opiate produced in the hypothalamus and in the brainstem, contributing to that delicious high you feel. This is the same hormone that diminishes pain levels. Prolactin, a chemical messenger responsible for more than 300 functions, gives you that relaxed sensation, and oxytocin promotes feelings of affection and triggers that nurturing instinct. Yes, it's the same bonding hormone that got pumped out of your brain alongside prolactin after you gave birth to turn your breasts on for feeding (and dare we say energizing) your newborn.

Exactly how these hormones affect sexual desire, arousal, and pleasure is an active area of research, but what is known so far is that all three hormones are released during orgasm and the net effect is satisfaction and contentment. And it's no surprise that your relaxed state of mind and body allow you to fall asleep rather quickly.

The message, in short: sex makes you look good and feel good. But you hopefully knew that from experience. If you don't feel like you're getting enough (and, like sleep, you know when you're deprived), this is something you'll want to address in your life.

Not in a relationship? Then go for the next best thing and treat yourself to more touching through massage. It may seem like a luxury, but it doesn't have to be. If you were to add up the cost of eating dinner out once a week for a month, you'd have plenty of money to get a massage, body scrub, and/or facial and enjoy all the amenities offered at most spas. The healing power of touch is grossly underestimated in our society, yet it's one of the most effective tools for emotional care.

I learned how valuable touch is to the energy of your spirit. I believe humans need and crave touch so powerfully, much more so than we know. A simple gesture communicates love, adoration, positivity, and a sense of value. My mother, my grandmother, my friends, have all taught me the beauty of a hug, a hand hold, a squeeze on the arm, a touch on the cheek. Physically showing love and concern towards your children is so important to their psyches. My grandmother used to always hug me, hold my hand, touch my hair and I knew she adored me. It made me feel alive in some special way. Sometimes we fear that touch will make us feel awkward and vulnerable so we shy away from it, but we shouldn't. It makes me sad when I see children not getting affection from their parents, or couples coexisting without touch and affection.

—VERONICA BOSGRAAF,
Pure Bar founder and mother

Massage not only benefits the muscles and tissues being kneaded and stretched but also has been found to lower stress levels significantly. It's been shown to increase weight gain in premature infants, alleviate depression, reduce pain in cancer patients, improve sleep patterns, and positively alter the immune system. Research from the renowned Touch Research Institute shows that it's as beneficial to touch as it is to be touched. And, more recently, researchers at the University of North Carolina, alongside scientists in Europe, are unraveling how the body responds to pleasurable touch. They have identified a class of nerve fibers in the skin that specifically send pleasure messages. Called the C-tactile nerve fibers, they send feel-good messages to the brain upon stimulation through pleasurable touch.

Healing touch therapy can take many forms, not just classic massage. Experiment with what your local spa has to offer. Bring this concept to home and into the bedroom with your partner, too. In between the more elaborate spa visits, schedule brief, inexpensive manicures, pedicures, or simply exchange five minutes of chair massage with your best friend at work. Studies have shown that these can dramatically reduce job stress while increasing productivity and alertness.

Be consistent. Make personal playtime a consistent habit. The key is to be sure the practice entails no phones, no talking, no way to be pulled back into the vortex of daily life, and it must be something doable on a regular basis. If you fluctuate ("I'll get a massage this week and go the movies with a girlfriend next week, etc.") then you're more apt to lose the habit. And lose your sanity. Having a consistent habit that's relaxing allows you to go into deeper relaxation every time.

Take action. Today, pick just one single habit you want to change and make a commitment to making that happen. It can be an ambitious goal such as quitting smoking or a small one such as reducing your consumption of fast food or replacing butter with extra-virgin olive oil in your cooking.

The Ten Essential Nutrients . . . they aren't found in food, but have everything to do with what food you choose and how your body uses it.

1. Nutrient L—for LAUGHTER . . .

2. Nutrient M—for MASSAGE . . .

3. Nutrient N—for NURTURE (YOURSELF as well as OTHERS) . . .

4. Nutrient O—for OXYGEN . . .

5. Nutrient P—for PHYSICAL ACTIVITY . . .

6. Nutrient Q—for QUIET . . .

7. Nutrient R—for RELAXATION . . .

8. Nutrient S—for SLEEP . . .

9. Nutrient T—for TIME . . .

10. Nutrient U—for UNDERSTANDING . . .

Take time to see where these nutrients fit into your plan. We promise, they make a huge difference

Source: Exceprted from Ashley's *Recipes for IBS: Great-Tasting Recipes and Tips Customized for Your Symptoms* (Fair Winds Press, 2007)

REFRESHED AND REJUVENATED

We hope that you understand the importance of play in your life. It's not something just for children. When you think about it, do you know anyone who comes back from a playful vacation complaining of exhaustion? Even if the vacation was physically demanding, the time away from the demands of everyday life was invigorating. But finding time to play needn't require two weeks off a year—or even a whole day to yourself. It can entail smaller, little pockets of time that you use to just exhale for a moment and recharge. It can be as simple as a 10-minute massage, or a movie night with friends or a loved one once a week. And it's not so much about finding time as it is about *making* time. All of us are overscheduled. The ones who can move meetings and commitments around to accommodate playtime are the happier survivors of that overscheduled life.

Mom Up! Jump-Start Your Transformation

Right this moment, take out your calendar—the thing you use to organize and schedule your life. Maybe it's all on your cell phone or perhaps you keep a traditional calendar on your wall at home. However you plan out your days, weeks, and months, now is the time to plan your playtime over the next 30 days. Pick at least one day a week (that's four times over the next month) when you carve out at least one hour for play (this doesn't include playtime with your kids, the bedtime hour, or even sex time; make this playtime totally separate and all about you minus the demands of everyday life). See if you can fill that one hour with something fun, such as lunch with a friend, a manicure or pedicure, or a dinner date with your spouse without the kids. Every month, when you pull out your calendar to plan ahead, see if you can plan your playtime in advance. The added challenge: try to find more than an hour here and there to play. Go away for a long weekend when the opportunity presents itself. Make a deposit on a vacation 6 to 12 months in advance so you don't let the whole year go by without a serious time-out.

The Choice Is Yours

Health is dynamic. Energy is, too. In either case, you don't get to achieve it and cross it off your list. It's like becoming a mom. You give your energy to your child from day one and then you're a mom forever . . . giving your energy away. You're a mom forever. You'll never get to be done with seeking optimal health throughout your life. But that's just life!

For many moms, it seems that your ability to choose is a window that is not as wide open as it used to be before giving birth. But it can be as wide open as you want it if you plan and choose carefully. Just as you chose to be a mom, you can choose to live your life a certain way that optimizes your energy and health. It's ultimately up to you to learn what makes you tick and feel fulfilled with that steady flow of energy. It may mean getting up at 5:30 to hop on a stationary bicycle, but then you're done with your exercise and don't have to think about it the rest of the day. You have a choice whether or not to plan at the top of the week and know what's coming down the pipeline. Are you the carpool person this week? On which nights do you have more time to cook? Can you find a night to go out with your husband or girlfriends? What after-school events require your attendance? When will you fit in your gardening? If you choose to lay back and say, "Can someone pick up the kids . . . and where's the pizza?" you'll pay consequences.

Of course, there will be things that go by the wayside, such as perfect nails and hair. In the long run, though, aren't you okay with that? Yes, because you get the important stuff done that ensures a healthy, happy family. And an energized mom who is ready to take on anything.

Final Note

By now we hope you've gained not only a lot of information on ways to improve your energy, but also a greater appreciation for your health and happiness. Your energy is not a fiction, just as Mom Energy is not an oxymoron. We applaud you in your decision to take better care of yourself, no matter how small a step you take starting today. Just picking up this book gives you points! And as you no doubt understand through personal experience alone, how energetic you feel says so much about you—your confidence, your courage, your character, and even your faith in yourself and the world at large.

Our knowledge about this astonishing link between our bodies and its myriad energy equations will only continue to expand. What we will discover in the future will reinforce the necessity to honor time-tested techniques for reducing and managing stress and choosing to maintain better lifestyles that can support our longevity. Remember, we want to live healthfully for as long as possible. Feeling as naturally energetic as possible in those later years ain't bad, either.

Your dedication to nurturing your body from an energy standpoint will reward you in so many fantastic ways—not just today, but every day forward for the rest of your life. We wish you the best of luck in your journey and encourage you to come back to this book when you need reminders about healthy, energetic living.

The Whole-Body List of Top Exercises

We realize it would be unwise of us to not at least give some specifics to working the body. Again, this is not meant to be a particular program. We just want to give you some of the tried-and-true methods of working the body that minimize your time commitment and maximize energy-generating results. These are great exercises to have on hand when you can't get to the gym or schedule a more formal workout. You'll find that many of these moves can be done in the comfort of your kitchen (while cooking) or den as you watch television and babysit a toddler playing nearby. All of them will pump your heart, get your blood running, and strengthen those little muscular engines that could! Added challenge: see if you can perform these exercises until you pant. Avoid performing the same routines on consecutive days, but try to incorporate all of them into your week, at least twice. Most of these exercises can be done in gyms using equipment, but they also can be done using props at home.

> **Caution:** Speak with your physician if you have specific health issues or physical limitations to contend with prior to commencing an exercise program, especially if you have not been active in a while. Your doctor can also help you gauge your fitness level and help you tailor an exercise program to your physical body. This will help lower your risk for injury or illness, as many people jump-start their fitness goals too quickly and wind up hurt and burned out. You must achieve a fine balance between pushing your body physically and staying attuned to its needs as you move forward.

LOWER BODY

Squat and Knee Lifts

There's a variety of ways to perform this one, but it's so versatile that you can be cooking in your kitchen and go through a couple of these heart pumpers. In a traditional squat and knee lift, you simply stand with feet hip distance apart and dip into a squat. In this position, your hips are back until your knees are bent to about a 90-degree angle. You can hold your hands in front of you around a small medicine ball or free weights. As you squat, sit back into your heels and keep your chest up. You don't want your knees to go in front of your toes. Then rise back up and lift one knee up until your upper leg is perpendicular to your body. Lower the leg and then repeat the squat. When you rise up again, lift the opposite leg.

Lunge and Squat Combo

Instead of a static lunge (returning your forward foot back to the original position), you can do a walking lunge, with a squat in between each step. So you lunge forward with the right foot and then take the left foot up to meet the right foot, then do a front squat. Repeat the sequence on the left side, lunging with the left foot forward, etc. Try making this a walking exercise, and watch your heart start pumping at a higher notch. Can you reach a point where you're starting to pant?

Toe and Hip Lift Hold *(or, How to Be Nice to Your Back and Work Your Butt Off!)*

Use a mat or cushioned floor. This exercise will relieve tension in your lower back and work your butt at the same time. Lie on your back with your arms at your sides with your knees bent and your feet on the floor. Lift your hips toward the ceiling, lifting your feet up on your toes. Hold for 1 count, and then lower back down. Repeat the lifts for 60 seconds, squeezing your glutes and hamstrings at the top of the range of motion. Be careful not to overarch your spine. For an added challenge, extend one leg at the top of the lift. Keep your thighs parallel and hold the lifted position for about 5 seconds. Keeping your hips up, place your foot back on the floor and then lower your hips. Repeat this exercise for 30 seconds; switch sides and do the move for another 30 seconds on the other leg.

Standing Single Leg Lifts

Ideally, this exercise should be done with a stability ball, a giant inflatable ball that you'll find at a sporting goods store or gym. This exercise will work the hip and thigh area. If you don't have access to a ball, try using the back of a chair. What you want to do is balance your weight on one leg while leaning on the exercise ball (or a chair).

To start, place the stability ball on the floor in front of you. Bend at the waist and place both hands shoulder width apart on the stability ball. Have a comfortable distance between your legs and the ball so you can bend comfortably. Your back should be parallel to the floor. Remember to maintain correct posture with a straight back and aligned shoulders; also make sure to place your head in alignment with your spine. Keeping your right foot on the ground, bend your right knee slightly and extend your left leg behind you until it is parallel with the floor. Your lifting leg should be in alignment with the rest of your body. Keep your foot flexed as you lift and tuck in your abdomen. Hold your lifted leg in position for 1 to 2 seconds and return it to the floor. Perform 10 repetitions for each leg. You can increase to 2 to 3 sets of standing leg lifts as your strength improves.

Double Stair Climb

It's proven that climbing stairs two at a time has tremendous advantages over taking one step at a time. When researchers at Pennsylvania State University in 2010 compared the metabolic cost and muscular activity of these two techniques, they found that, indeed, skipping a step leads to a measurable difference in energy usage. Translation: your body will burn more energy, which then cycles back to infuse you with more energy. Case closed.

Find a good set of stairs in your neighborhood, hopefully one that has more than 10 steps, but anything will do. Get into a rhythm of climbing 2 steps at a time, and then walk back down 1 step at a time. Repeat. See if you can go for at least 15 minutes. Vary the speed—you can start by walking, then ramp up your speed to a semi-run or a full-fledged run. Given your comfort level and the depth/size of the stairs, you can also try to walk down the staircase two at a time, or pick up your downstep pace, too. Moving in both directions will pump your heart and give you a great lower-body workout.

Wall Sit with Leg Crossed

Stand in front of a wall (about 2 feet in front of it) and lean against it. Slide down until your knees are at about 90-degree angles and hold, keeping the abs contracted. Find your stability, and then cross one leg over the other. Relax your arms, keep your chest open, and shoulders back against the wall. Hold for as long as you can, about 15 seconds to a minute. Then switch legs, crossing the other and holding. Do 2 or 3 rounds.

CORE

Plank

Lie facedown on a mat or a carpeted floor, resting on your forearms with palms flat on the floor. Push off the floor, raising up onto toes and resting on the elbows. Keep your back flat, in a straight line from head to heels. Tilt your pelvis and contract your abdominals to prevent your rear end from sticking up in the air or sagging in the middle. Hold for 20 to 60 seconds, lower, and repeat for 3 to 5 reps.

On-Your-Side Hip Lift

Lie on your left side with legs extended, right leg slightly in front of the left, body weight supported on your left elbow and left hip. Your right arm rests on your right side, and your left elbow is bent and in line with your left shoulder, palm on floor.

Contract your abs and hold your torso erect; it should form a straight line between your head and your hips. Using your left upper-hip and buttocks muscles and keeping your abs tight, press the side of your left foot into the floor and lift your hips until your body forms a straight line from head to feet. Hold for a count of 3, and then lower your hips to the starting position. Complete 10 reps and switch sides. Do 3 sets on each side. Bonus: perform the last set on one leg by lifting your top leg off the floor and holding it in line with and just above your bottom leg.

Flat-Arm Crunch

The flat-, or long-arm, crunch is sixth in the list of top 10 most effective abdominal exercises. It's been proven to produce 19 percent more muscle activity than a traditional crunch. As with any abdominal exercise, the flat-arm crunch relies on slow, controlled movements. The abdominal muscles should be tightened or engaged in order to make the upper body move. Properly done, this exercise requires very little movement up and off of the floor. Consistent abdominal pressure is the key to this movement.

Lie flat on your back with your knees bent and the feet flat on the floor. Extend your arms above and slightly behind the head (not bent—they remain extended, or "flat"). Your hands should be held close together. Contract your abdominals and bring your shoulder blades off the floor. Then lower your body back down to the starting point. Repeat for at least 20 counts. See if you can do 3 sets of 20.

During the exercise, the arms should remain next to the ears. They should not fall forward and away from the head. The reason for this is to limit the extent to which other muscle groups, other than the abdominals, are used. Throwing the arms forward can grant extra momentum, undermining the effectiveness of the movement. Similarly, straining with the neck or head to raise the trunk of the body should be avoided.

Jump and Touch

Find an object about 18 inches above your tiptoe reach. It can be a bar, the top of a doorframe, or a 5-pound ring you dangle from a doorframe. Jump straight up into the air, touching the object at the peak of the jump. Avoid going into a full squat before each jump. Make sure you can tap the object each time you jump. Try 3 sets of 20 jumps each.

UPPER BODY

Triceps Dips with Straight Legs

Sit on a chair or step. Grasp the front edge of the seat near the thighs. Walk feet forward until hips are slightly bent, legs straight, arms extended (don't lock the elbows). Keep feet hip-width apart. Bend elbows about 90 degrees and lower hips toward the floor. Inhale as you go down. If you feel pain in the shoulders, your elbows are bent too much. As you exhale, press up until elbows are straight, but not locked. Repeat this action 15 to 20 times. Go 3 rounds.

Triceps Dips with One Leg Crossed

Perform the same action as above, but cross one leg over the other. After a round of 15 to 20 dips, switch legs and repeat. Go 3 rounds on each leg.

Push-up

Assume the traditional push-up position on the floor: palms of hands flat on floor slightly more than shoulder width apart; legs straight, with weight on balls of the feet; feet just a few inches apart. If you find this exercise too difficult, you may modify the basic position by having your knees, rather than the balls of your feet, touch the floor. Inhale as you lower your body to the floor; exhale as you lift it. Repeat 15 to 20 times in succession. If doing 2 sets, rest for no more than 30 seconds between sets.

The following exercises require free weights. Get yourself a pair of dumbbells that are comfortable to hold. You're likely to want to increase the weights as you get stronger, so start with a set of 3-pounders and add more as you go. Work up to using 8- and 10-pounders in each hand.

Shoulder Presses

Sit on the end of a bench or use a bench/chair that supports the back. Hold dumbbells in each hand. Hold weights with palms facing out and elbows at 90 degrees, palms at shoulder level.

As you exhale, push weights overhead until arms are straight and in line with shoulders. Don't lock elbows completely. Then, as you inhale, return to starting position to complete 1 rep. Perform 15 to 20 reps, and go for 3 rounds.

Bicep Curls

Stand with feet slightly apart, knees slightly bent, and abs tight. Grasp a dumbbell in each hand with an underhand grip. Lock elbows into the side of your torso and rest weights in your hands, on the front of your thighs. As you inhale, curl one dumbbell to your shoulder. Then, exhale and lower dumbbell to starting position; then curl the dumbbell in your opposite hand.

One curl on each side equals 1 rep. Perform 15 to 20 reps, and go for 3 rounds. (Note: Keeping abs tight will help protect your lower back. If your body leans backward as you curl up the weight, then the weight is too heavy. Keep elbows pressed into your sides for support and to isolate the biceps. This exercise can also be done in a seated position.)

Bicep Curl with Squat

This will get your upper and lower body working simultaneously. With your feet shoulder-width apart, hold the dumbbells by your side. Squat back as if you're going to sit on a chair, and perform a bicep curl on the way up. Inhale on the way down, and exhale on the way up.

Acknowledgments

As with all books, it takes a small army of talented, bright, and energetic people to weave together a manuscript worthy of publication. This one is no different. We owe everyone we've ever worked with through the years a heartfelt thank you, especially the mothers who've been the inspiration for this book. The unwavering support of our families, friends, colleagues, and clients have also paved the path to this book. Your guidance, insights, and feedback were indispensible; *Mom Energy* is as much yours as it is ours.

Collectively we'd like to express our gratitude to the many extraordinary people who trained their efforts on this project from start to finish. To those who provided tips and offered comments, and to the moms who allowed us to quote their remarks, we thank you.

To our indefatigable agent, Laurie Bernstein, who went beyond the call of duty and orchestrated so much of our creative energy when the initial concepts were just beginning to germinate in the proposal phase. You provided the roadmap for this book, and your unwavering support from day one has been invaluable. Thanks to Laurie, we met our talented writer, Kristin Loberg, who took our voice, thoughts, and ideas to the page. You inspire us with your blind plunge into a "mom" project, and during the process became one yourself.

To the team at Hay House, who endured all of our last-minute requests and changes, and whose insights helped produce the best book possible. Thanks especially to Patty Gift, Laura Koch, Sally Mason, Reid Tracy, Margarete Nielsen, Gail Gonzales, Carina Sammartino, and all the other wonderful, hard-working souls at Hay House.

Thank you to Lisa Fyfe for your creative genius and willingness to go the distance.

And now, to a few more individuals that each of us would like to call out:

From Ashley:

So many people contributed to this book, and I thank them for their energy and their role in enabling mine. I thank the team on this book—"the *Mom Energy* gals"—including my co-author, Kathy, an exceptionally talented individual and friend. All of you have shown me that *Mom Energy* has so many different presentations, each of them beautiful, respectful, funny, and inspiring.

To the women in my life: Mom, Irma, Camille, Juliet, my friends, and their moms, too. They support my energy by giving the gifts of example, suggestions, and never-ending encouragement for which I am grateful beyond words. I also thank the men in my life: Dad, Corey, Jon, and Austin. All of you are *Mom Energy* enablers in different ways, and I admire each of you for your unique blend of humor and compassion.

I thank my energy team: Doron, Dr. DG, Brad, Ben, Jason, my agent Amy Stanton, my publicists Melinda and Ryan, and the AKA team: Matthew H. and Matt T., Amy F. and Rerun. Thank you for being there for me and for nurturing my body, voice, and spirit.

From Kathy:

I would love to say that my energy allows me to do it all, but I've had an extra set of hands for many years, and I would like to thank Kathleen Ingle for helping me keep up the pace that I have grown accustomed to.

Thanks to my longtime publicist, Sharon House, whose support through the years eventually led to this important book.

And of course, a special thanks goes to my comrade and tireless book partner, Ashley. Had it not been for your tenacity, enthusiasm, and collaborative wisdom on nutrition and energy metabolism, this book might never have gotten to where it needed to be.

I have great respect for women who take the journey of motherhood, a journey that is sprinkled with trials and tribulations. I could not have found reason to write this book had it not been for my mom and my children.

Finally, I'd like to personally extend another round of applause to all the moms in the world. We are one in the love of our children.

About the Authors

Ashley Koff, R.D., is a registered dietitian with the proven ability to demystify the science of nutrition and communicate the importance of a healthy lifestyle to clients in a way that instills loyalty and trust.

Named among the Top 10 Registered Dietitians in the U.S. by *Today's Dietitian* magazine and Best of LA's "Nutritionist/Dietitians" by *Citysearch* three years running, Koff appears regularly on national media outlets, including *The Dr. Oz Show, The Doctors,* CBS's *The Early Show, Good Morning America Health,* CNN, AOL, and E!; and was the lead expert for *The Huffington Post Living's* "Total Energy Makeover with Ashley Koff RD." Koff is frequently featured in national publications such as *The New York Times, InStyle, Reader's Digest, Every Day with Rachael Ray, Redbook, Women's Health, Shape,* and *O, The Oprah Magazine.* She is a contributing editor for *Natural Health* magazine, the dietitian for espnW, and a member of the advisory board of *Fitness* magazine. Koff has been the featured dietitian on the CW's couples health transformation show, *Shedding for the Wedding,* and Lifetime's *Love Handles.* In 2007, she authored *Recipes for IBS,* a cookbook and treatment plan for digestive wellness.

As part of her "Qualitarian" mission, Koff is committed to helping consumers, health-care practitioners, and the media easily identify products that contribute to a healthy lifestyle. At her nutrition counseling and consulting company, she created The Ashley Koff Approved (AKA) Lists, a tool to help people identify products that meet a high standard of nutrition and marketing integrity. Curiosity and a desire to get the whole story on food ingredients, Koff routinely "goes to the source" around the world and throughout the U.S. to explore food production and cultural influences in our food system.

Koff maintains a private practice, regularly lectures, is a spokesperson for several national brands, and works to improve the quality of food choices in numerous outlets including on the sets of popular shows like ABC's *Private Practice,* CBS's *CSI: New York,* HBO's *Big Love,* FX's *It's Always Sunny in Philadelphia,* and FOX's *Bones.*

Educated at both Duke and New York Universities, Koff trained at LA+USC and Columbus Children's hospitals and also worked at Cedars-Sinai Medical Center in Los Angeles.

Website: **www.AshleyKoffRD.com**

Kathy Kaehler has devoted her life to helping people live happy, productive, and healthy lives as an author, celebrity trainer, spokesperson, and mom. She is a National Fitness Hall of Famer and continues to shape the bodies and inspire the lives of millions around the world.

For 13 years, she appeared on the *Today* show's exercise segments with Katie Couric, Matt Lauer, and Ann Curry. She has worked out with numerous A-list celebrities including Julia Roberts, Michelle Pfeiffer, Cindy Crawford, Jennifer Aniston, Drew Barrymore, Jennifer Lopez, Denise Richards, Claudia Schiffer, and Kim Basinger. Her work with Kim Kardashian in 2009 led to a downloadable workout series and added yet another DVD video—*Kim Kardashian's Body Beautiful*—to Kathy's large collection.

As a prolific and best-selling author, Kaehler has written many books, including *Teenage Fitness, Fit and Sexy for Life,* and *Kathy Kaehler's Celebrity Workouts.* She has been a contributing writer to *Elle, Self,* and *Women's Sports and Fitness* and her workouts and training tips have appeared in *InStyle, Us Weekly, Shape, Fitness, Family Circle, Health, More, Allure, Marie Claire,* and *Woman's Day,* among many others. Kathy was a regular contributor to MSNBC. com and wrote biweekly columns for the *Los Angeles Daily News,* which was syndicated to several other major markets. In addition to the *Today* show, Kathy has appeared on such shows as *The View, The Megan Mullally Show, The Best Damn Sports Show,* and *The Oprah Winfrey Show.*

As an in-demand spokesperson, Kathy has worked with a number of brands and products including Boniva, Healthy Ones, Hanes, Propel, Vaseline, Nasonex, Ragu, the Milk Board, Chilean Fresh Fruit, MIO watches, Walkmill portable treadmill, Serta, Breyers, and Enell bras. Kathy is currently the leading health and fitness spokesperson for USANA and creator of Sunday Set-Up™. She also is a Podfitness Premiere Trainer and one of the stars of Lifetime's *My Workout.*

Kaehler believes that everyone, at any age, should adopt a lifestyle that incorporates fitness, good nutrition, and a positive outlook. As a mother to three boys—15-year-old twins and an 11-year old—she knows about Mom Energy.

Website: **www.kathykaehler.net**

HAY HOUSE TITLES
OF RELATED INTEREST

YOU CAN HEAL YOUR LIFE, the movie,
starring Louise L. Hay & Friends
(available as a 1-DVD program and an expanded 2-DVD set)
Watch the trailer at: **www.LouiseHayMovie.com**

THE SHIFT, the movie,
starring Dr. Wayne W. Dyer
(available as a 1-DVD program and an expanded 2-DVD set)
Watch the trailer at: **www.DyerMovie.com**

A COURSE IN WEIGHT LOSS:
21 Spiritual Lessons for Surrendering Your Weight Forever,
by Marianne Williamson

ARE YOU TIRED AND WIRED?:
*Your Proven 30-Day Program for Overcoming
Adrenal Fatigue and Feeling Fantastic Again,*
by Marcelle Pick, MSN, OB/GYN NP

FRIED:
Why You Burn Out and How to Revive,
by Joan Borysenko, Ph.D.

WISHES FOR A MOTHER'S HEART:
Words of Inspiration, Love, and Support,
by Tricia LaVoice and Barbara Lazaroff

All of the above are available at your local bookstore,
or may be ordered by contacting Hay House (see next page).

We hope you enjoyed this Hay House book. If you'd like to receive our online catalog featuring additional information on Hay House books and products, or if you'd like to find out more about the Hay Foundation, please contact:

Hay House, Inc., P.O. Box 5100, Carlsbad, CA 92018-5100
(760) 431-7695 or (800) 654-5126
(760) 431-6948 (fax) or (800) 650-5115 (fax)
www.hayhouse.com® • **www.hayfoundation.org**

Published and distributed in Australia by:
Hay House Australia Pty. Ltd., 18/36 Ralph St., Alexandria NSW 2015 •
Phone: 612-9669-4299 • *Fax:* 612-9669-4144 • www.hayhouse.com.au

Published and distributed in the United Kingdom by:
Hay House UK, Ltd., 292B Kensal Rd., London W10 5BE •
Phone: 44-20-8962-1230 • *Fax:* 44-20-8962-1239 • www.hayhouse.co.uk

Published and distributed in the Republic of South Africa by:
Hay House SA (Pty), Ltd., P.O. Box 990, Witkoppen 2068
Phone/Fax: 27-11-467-8904 • www.hayhouse.co.za

Published in India by:
Hay House Publishers India, Muskaan Complex, Plot No. 3, B-2,
Vasant Kunj, New Delhi 110 070 • *Phone:* 91-11-4176-1620
Fax: 91-11-4176-1630 • www.hayhouse.co.in

Distributed in Canada by:
Raincoast, 9050 Shaughnessy St.,
Vancouver, B.C. V6P 6E5 • *Phone:* (604) 323-7100
Fax: (604) 323-2600 www.raincoast.com

Take Your Soul on a Vacation

Visit **www.HealYourLife.com®** to regroup, recharge,
and reconnect with your own magnificence.
Featuring blogs, mind-body-spirit news, and life-changing
wisdom from Louise Hay and friends.

Visit **www.HealYourLife.com** today!